Female Genital Mutilation

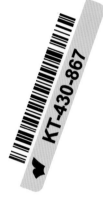

BMA

Edited by

Comfort Momoh

Forewords by

Dame Karlene Davis

and

Christine McCafferty

Radcliffe Publishing
Oxford • Seattle

Radcliffe Publishing Ltd
18 Marcham Road
Abingdon
Oxon OX14 1AA
United Kingdom

www.radcliffe-oxford.com
Electronic catalogue and worldwide online ordering facility.

© 2005 Comfort Momoh

British Library Cataloguing in Publication Data.

A catalogue record for this book is available from the British Library.

ISBN 1 85775 693 2

Typeset by Aarontype Ltd, Easton, Bristol
Printed and bound by TJ International Ltd, Padstow, Cornwall

Contents

Foreword

It is difficult to estimate the number of women across the world who may have suffered as a result of female genital mutilation (FGM). The World Health Organization has estimated numbers as high as 120 million women in more than 30 countries. There are no medical, hygiene or health reasons for women to be subjected to FGM, but it persists as a deep-rooted traditional practice in many African and Middle Eastern countries.

Although FGM is an illegal practice in the UK, some women who have arrived in Britain as refugees or migrants from other countries, may have been subjected to the procedure in one form or another.

As midwives, we need to be able to provide a high quality service to all the women for whom we care. As professionals, we need to be aware of the impact of FGM on a woman's reproductive experience and work to meet these women's needs, both in terms of clinical care and emotional support.

Unfortunately, because of the nature of FGM, there has sometimes been a lack of guidelines and research for professionals caring for these women. This book bridges that gap, and provides advice for midwives and other health professionals on how to improve the reproductive health and childbirth experiences of women who have suffered FGM.

The Royal College of Midwives is committed to supporting midwives in understanding that, although the practice of FGM is illegal in the UK, women who have experienced this are a part of contemporary British society, and may therefore require the care of a midwife at some point in their lives.

I am delighted to recommend this book to you and hope that it will equip you with the tools to continue to care for women with compassion and with confidence.

Dame Karlene Davis DBE
General Secretary
The Royal College of Midwives
September 2005

Foreword

Female genital mutilation (FGM), also known as female genital cutting or female circumcision, involves procedures which include the partial or total removal of the external female genital organs for cultural or other non-therapeutic reasons.

The issues raised by FGM are many and complex. Four main justifications are cited for this harmful practice, namely custom/tradition, religion, social pressure and women's sexuality. Although these four justifications exist for the maintenance of the practice, it appears to be linked primarily to a desire to subordinate women and to control their sexuality.

The United Nations General Assembly has adopted several resolutions calling on governments to eradicate FGM, and some countries have passed legislation to ban and criminalise the practice. FGM violates the reproductive rights and human rights of women and girls because it interferes with their right to bodily integrity by removing their healthy sexual organs without medical necessity. FGM violates the rights to non-discrimination, health and bodily integrity.

Although FGM is not undertaken with the intention of inflicting harm, its damaging physical, sexual and psychological effects make it an act of violence against women and children. FGM sometimes threatens the lives of girls and women, thereby violating their human rights to life, liberty and security of the person. FGM is a violation of children's rights because FGM is commonly performed upon girls between the ages of four and twelve, who are not in a position to give informed consent.

Governments must undertake efforts at the community level to inform women of the health risks of FGM. Additionally, the Convention on the Rights of the Child, the Convention on the Elimination of All Forms of Discrimination Against Women, and recommendations of the Committee on the Elimination of Discrimination Against Women explicitly recognise harmful traditional practices such as FGM as violations of human rights. In addition, women and children who have already been subjected to FGM and who are suffering from the complications of the procedure should have access to the care they need.

Because enabling women to make the choice to abandon FGM requires an improvement of women's status, governments should reform all existing laws that serve as barriers to women's equality. In many cases, this requires changing family laws, such as those that relate to marriage, divorce, child custody, inheritance, as well as laws relating to property. Women cannot stand alone in their demand for social justice. They must involve other sectors of society. Women need allies among politicians, religious leaders, health professionals and all other influential individuals and groups in society.

In 1994 Ghana became the first African nation to outlaw FGM. It was followed by Burkina Faso, Côte d'Ivoire and Senegal. Uganda adopted a new constitution in 1995, which states that, 'Laws, cultures, customs or traditions, which are against the dignity, welfare or interest of women or which undermine their status are prohibited by this constitution'. In Uganda a project has greatly reduced the incidence of FGM by separating the practice itself from the cultural values it was intended to support and by proposing alternative activities to sustain those ideals.

In the UK, the Female Circumcision Act came into force on 16 July 1985, and made FGM illegal in the country. There have been no prosecutions under this law so far, however. In 2000 the UK All Party Parliamentary Group on Population, Development and Reproductive Health held Parliamentary Hearings on FGM. As a follow-up to the Hearings at the beginning of the 2002–03 parliamentary session the FGM Bill was debated in both chambers and passed with all party consensus, gaining Royal Assent on 23 October 2003.

The new FGM law extends to extra-territorial acts. The person assisting will be guilty under the Act and can be liable on conviction on indictment, to imprisonment for a term of up to 14 years or a fine (or both). The new FGM Act can be viewed in detail on the web at www.hmso.gov.uk/acts/acts2003/20030031.htm.

Legislation alone will not eradicate the practice but the aim of strengthening the law in this way is to send a strong message about the unacceptability of the FGM and to hopefully have a deterrent effect. It will provide a useful springboard for taking forward the wider enforcement and education activities in consultation and collaboration with NGOs and social and health professionals.

FGM is a barbaric attack on women's sexuality and autonomy. We must all – politicians, clinicians, community and religious leaders – join together to ensure that FGM is eradicated both in the UK and abroad. FGM is a fundamental human rights issue with adverse health and social implications. FGM violates the rights of girls and women to bodily integrity and results in perpetuating gender inequality.

It is vital that FGM laws are fully implemented and that governments, agencies, professionals and communities work together for the elimination of this practice.

Chris McCafferty

Christine McCafferty MP
Chair, UK All Party Parliamentary Group on Population,
Development and Reproductive Health
September 2005

Preface

Female genital mutilation (FGM) or female circumcision is a growing problem in the UK and Europe among African community and asylum seekers. There are an increasing number of asylum seekers entering UK and Europe; for example, in the UK in 2001, approximately 17 720 applications were received at Quarter 4 and 22 760 in same quarter in 2002. Of these, a significant number are from countries still practising FGM.

Many women are still being re-sewn (infibulated) by doctors and midwives following childbirth. On occasions, women are undergoing unnecessary Caesarean section. About 75% of health and social care professionals are still not aware of the legal issues surrounding FGM and how to protect children at risk of FGM. Practitioners in the UK now face dilemmas and complexities of understanding the practice, as well as providing adequate appropriate holistic care to this group of vulnerable women and girls.

Very little factual information is available in the UK for health professionals and those working in a lay capacity with voluntary and community organisations. Pre-existing text on the subject is largely outdated and the context within which it was written does not lend itself to current health promotion practices, current changes in health and healthcare provision, changes to nurses and medical curriculum and the recent changes to legislation.

Every month I am contacted by, on average, 15 to 20 students or professionals wishing to share information and support guidelines, to inform knowledge and practice and, as an educational strategy, to seek elective placement. By focusing on this specialist issue, this book provides an excellent resource, thus reducing considerably the one-to-one work that is currently done both at national and inter-national level and raising awareness of the subject concerning the socio-cultural, ethical-legal, sexual health and clinical implications of FGM.

Health and social care professionals are in need of factual, up-to-date and user-friendly information. This text will encourage the reader to grasp the fundamental principles of FGM within a cultural context and provide a practical approach to reducing mental and physical harm. The book will be a resource for health professionals at all levels including nursing, midwifery and medical practitioners.

Health promoters, practice nurses and health visitors will also benefit from the practical nature of the text. It will inform practice, policies and guidelines and be useful for informing the knowledge of student midwives, health promoters, prac-tice nurses, health visitors and doctors during their training and those studying for Certificate, Diploma and Master's degree.

Lay members of organisations working in the community, with special interest in the issue of FGM, will find the book a useful point of reference and it is envisaged that it will be a key text on the reading list for medical and non-medical curriculum courses.

Please note that the females depicted on the front cover have not been circumcised.

Comfort Momoh
September 2005

About the author

Comfort Momoh is an FGM Consultant/Public Health Specialist, with extensive experience of holistic women-centred care management, who conducts research into women's health and is a strong campaigner for the eradication of Female Genital Mutilation (FGM).

Comfort established and runs the African Well Woman's Clinic at Guy's and St Thomas' Foundation Trust, a support service for women and girls who have undergone FGM, and she became the first ever Nurse/Midwife of the Year at Guy's and St Thomas' Foundation Trust in 2003. She also received merit at the Nursing Times award in 2003 and she holds a Masters degree from the University of London.

Comfort is an expert in the field of FGM and her work is well known to healthcare professionals and NGOs throughout the United Kingdom, Europe and worldwide. She provides counselling, advice, support and information and performs surgical reversal of FGM in her clinic and prides herself on being able to make a difference to the lives of the often vulnerable people she cares for.

Comfort also provides training and runs workshops, seminars and conferences at local, national and international level. Comfort has served as a temporary consultant with the World Health Organization, is Chairperson for Black Women's Health and Family Support (a non-governmental organisation working with and supporting the community); she is also the Vice President for EuroNet (European Network on FGM).

Comfort is happily married with two daughters and lives in North London.

List of contributors

Marwa Ahmed
Conducted research at Southampton University with assistance from Mr RW Stones, Consultant Obs & Gynae at Princess Ann Hospital, Southampton and Senior Lecturer at Southampton University

Jacqueline Dunkley-Bent MSc ADM, PGCEA, RM, RGN, MRIPH
Counsellor in Rape and Sexual Assault, Consultant Midwife – Public Health and Head of Midwifery job share, Guy's and St Thomas' NHS Trust

Harry Gordon FRCS (Edinburgh), FRCOG
The African Clinic, Central Middlesex Hospital

Adwoa Kwateng-Kluvitse
Director of FORWARD

Els Leye
Senior Project Manager, International Centre for Reproductive Health, Ghent University

Sarah McCulloch
National Director, Agency for Culture and Change Management, Sheffield

Sadiya Mohammad BSc (Hons) International Health

Janice Rymer MD, FRCOG, FRANZCOG, ILTM
Professor of Obstetrics and Gynaecology at Guy's, King's and St Thomas' School of Medicine, Guy's and St Thomas' NHS Foundation Trust

Nahid Toubia MD BCH, FRCS (England)
President of Rainb♀, Health and Rights of African Women, London, UK

Dedication/acknowledgement

This book is dedicated to the millions of women and girls worldwide who have been circumcised. As a woman, specialist and expert in this field, I share your pain and burden; but I know that there is hope and light at the end of the tunnel and with the help of all well-meaning people worldwide your daughters will not have to undergo the same trauma and experience as you.

To all NGOs, local and international organisations, hospitals, PCTs, individuals, men and women, anthropologists and human rights activists who are campaigning tirelessly to eradicate FGM.

Gratitude goes to my husband Robert and daughters Flora and Laura for their support and encouragement in writing this book.

Introduction

In societies where female genital mutilation (FGM) prevails, one can see elements of culture that include particular beliefs, behavioural norms, customs, rituals, social hierarchies and religious, political and economic systems. Such communities share ways of living their lives and tend to think in the same way; however, culture is learnt and children learn culture from adults. FGM is supported by centuries of tradition, culture and false beliefs and is perpetuated by poverty, illiteracy, low status of women and inadequate healthcare facilities.[1–3]

FGM is linked to strongly held ideas about identity, sexuality, gender and power.[4] Women who have undergone FGM are said to be highly regarded within practising communities, those who do not have FGM performed being viewed as unable to become mature women, unaccepted in their community and unqualified for marriage and childbearing.[5]

United Nations International Children's Emergency Fund (UNICEF) describes FGM as a deeply rooted tradition that is perceived in many societies to be a religious obligation, in Africa and Arab Islamic countries in particular. However, Islamic scholars have delivered edicts, clearly stating that the practice of FGM is not obligatory in Islam; there is nothing in the Koran, or the Sunnah, to suggest that it is a prescribed ritual of initiation for women.[6] Mali is an example of a staunchly Islamic country, where organisations and progressive Imams are working together to spread the message that abandoning the custom of FGM is not a sin against Islam, but the end of a dangerous practice that can have long-lasting health repercussions.[7]

One has to understand the strong motivating factors that prevail in practising communities. These include the prospect of becoming a social outcast, rejection by peers and family and loss of security and support.[8,9] In certain groups, the greatest insult possible is to be referred to as the 'son of an uncircumcised woman'.[10] Marriage is the main means of survival and security in a patriarchal society where women have no autonomy, power, status or education.[11]

There are aspects of the issue of FGM on which most agree. There is a fundamental need to take a holistic perspective that embraces the rich, multifaceted and diverse tapestry that is Africa, the Middle East and Asia. Those who continue to perpetuate the practice of FGM defend it, proclaiming it as a gift they bestow on their female children. They find the implication that they are child abusers deeply offensive, arguing that the actual day of circumcision is one of accomplishment and recognition of a girl's rite of passage into womanhood.[12]

Debate about FGM often reveals a dichotomy – collective versus individual rights. Those opposed to the practice argue that individuals, both men and women, have right of autonomy and to enjoying a full range of human rights and freedoms. Those who defend the practice take the view that there must be respect for a person's particular cultural identity and that the rights of minorities must be protected.[13] An integrated approach must be informed by such philosophical values and beliefs, whilst making use of legal measures, outreach services and health promotion and education programmes.[14]

In the context of understanding people who come from such collectivist cultures, in the developing world, to take up residence in the West, where emphasis is more on individuality and self-sufficiency, one must realise that this can cause feelings of bewilderment and disorientation. In addressing the issue of FGM, it is important to identify and protect the needs of girls who have not yet been circumcised, whilst remaining conscious of the implications of change for the self-esteem of mothers.[15]

Throughout history and to the present day we can see graphic illustrations of people's desire to alter their bodies for reasons of beautification, cultural acceptance, respect for societal norms and obligation, actual or perceived, to religious dictum.[16] There has certainly been considerable debate as to whether Western nations are guilty of double standards and intolerance, citing instances of physical mutilation – body piercing, designer vaginas and breast implantation, for example – as illustrations of accepted practices that form part of a group or culture's identity.

Ogundipe-Leslie cites growing number of 'narratives of victimhood' about African women in Euro-American discourse that appear conveniently detached from the 'mutilation' inflicted on females during Western cosmetic surgery.[17] There are, however, several features of FGM that distinguish it from other forms of body modification. Such comparisons are suspect when one considers the severe risks and potentially life-threatening complications of FGM that are largely imposed on children who have no voice in the decision.

The age at which FGM is performed varies according to the country, tribe and circumstances, and ranges from a few days old to adolescence, adulthood, just before marriage or after the first pregnancy. Somalis tend to perform FGM on girls aged from four to nine years; the Ethiopian Falashas carry out the procedure when a baby is a few days old.[18] In Eastern Ethiopia, the Adere and Oromo groups perform FGM between four years of age and puberty, whilst in Amhara it is on the eighth day after birth.[19] Girls may be circumcised alone or with a group of peers from their community.[1]

This book has been written in anticipation that it will assist those of you who care about the health and well-being of women and girls who have had, or are at risk of having, FGM. This includes those of you working in the healthcare professions, social services, teaching, child protection agencies, the police service, caseworkers involved with refugees and asylum seekers, children's charities, non-governmental organisations (NGOs), policymakers and academics. We hope that whatever your discipline you will find the information helpful in exploring the complex issues surrounding this sensitive subject.

Contributors have made a great effort to stay objective and present a holistic picture of current situation. Our primary concern is for the health of those who are suffering the consequences of having undergone FGM and to safeguard and protect young women and girls who remain vulnerable to this practice. That said, we acknowledge that mothers who submit their daughters to this procedure do so, from their perspective, as an act of love and for the noblest of reasons.

Some readers will already have knowledge and expertise in this field, others will have come to hear about the practice recently; whichever is the case, we hope that by the time you have read the book you will have a better understanding of the historical, physical, psychosexual, socio-economic and cultural factors that underpin the maintenance of what is an ancient tradition. Most important of all, the authors earnestly hope that we have persuaded you to continue the journey with us, to put an end to this harmful ritualistic practice.

References

1   Dorkenoo E (1995) *Cutting the Rose. Female genital mutilation: the practice and its prevention.* Minority Rights Publications, London.
2   Allam MFA, de Irala-Estevez J, Navajas RF *et al.* (1999) Student's knowledge of and attitudes about female circumcision in Egypt. *NEJM.* **341**: 1552–3.
3   Eke N (2000) Female genital mutilation: what can be done? *Lancet.* **356**(Supplement): 57.
4   Rahman A and Toubia N (2000) *Female Genital Mutilation: a guide to the laws and policies.* Worldwide Zed Books, London.
5   Momoh C (2000) *Female Genital Mutilation: information for health care professionals.* King's Fund, London.
6   IslamOnline.net & News Agencies (February 7 2004) – First anniversary of the International Day of Zero Tolerance of Female Genital Mutilation and Cutting (female circumcision).
7   Afrol News (June 2004) FGM in Mali connected to pre-Islamic traditions. UN media IRIN.
8   Gibeau AM (1998) Female genital mutilation: when a cultural practice generates clinical and ethical dilemmas. *J Obstet Gynecol Neonatal Nurs.* **27**: 85–91.
9   Momoh C (1999) Female genital mutilation: the struggle continues. *Pract Nurs.* **10**: 31–3.
10 Lightfoot-Klein H (1989) *Prisoners of Ritual: an odyssey into female genital mutilation in Africa.* Haworth Press, New York.
11 Foundation for Women's Health Research and Development (FORWARD) (2000) *Factsheet: female genital mutilation.* FORWARD, London.
12 Iweriebor Ifeyinwa (1994) *Brief Reflections on Clitoridectomy.* BWP, New York.
13 Breitung B (1996) *Interpretation and Eradication: National and International Responses To Female Circumcision.* 10 Emory-Int'l. Rev. 657.
14 World Health Organization (2000) *Factsheet 241.* World Health Organization, Geneva.
15 Barnes-Dean V (1985) Clitoridectomy and infibulation. *Cultural Survival Quarterly.* **9.2**: 1–8.
16 Hellsten SK (2004) Rationalising circumcision: from tradition to fashion, from public health to individual freedom – critical notes on cultural persistence of the practice of genital mutilation. *Med Ethics.* **30**: 248–53.
17 Ogundipe-Leslie M (1994) *Recreating Ourselves: African women and critical transformations.* Africa World Press, Trenton, NJ.
18 Ng F (2000) Female genital mutilation: its implication for reproductive health. An overview. *Br J Fam Plan.* **26**: 47–51.
19 Missailidis K and Gebre-Medhin M (2000) Female genital mutilation declines in Ethiopia. *Lancet.* **356**: 137–8.

Chapter One

Female genital mutilation

Comfort Momoh

History

The history of ritual genital surgery on women is not well known, but the practice of FGM dates back at least 2000 years.[1,2] Herodotus mentions the custom specifically, informing us that Phoenicians, Hittites and Ethiopians, as well as the Egyptians, undertook the practice. Some authors believe that it was practised in ancient Egypt, as a sign of distinction among the aristocracy, and have reported that traces of infibulation can still be found on Egyptian mummies.[3]

At a point in history that is obscure, there was strong emphasis on the importance of women's virginity and virtue that still forms part of cultures in Africa and Arab nations today; this combination resulted in the radical practice of infibulation.[4] Greek physicians who visited Egypt described the procedure, explaining that its purpose was the reduction of female sexual desire caused by the enlargement of the clitoris from its rubbing on the women's clothing.[5]

Many commentators believe that the practice evolved from earliest times in primitive communities that wished to establish control over the sexual behaviour of women. The Romans performed a technique involving slipping of rings through the labia majora of female slaves to prevent them becoming pregnant[6] and the Scoptsi sect in Russia performed FGM to ensure virginity.[2]

FGM has existed in one form or another in almost all known civilisations throughout history and has not been confined to a particular culture or religion. FGM is usually to be found in a traditional group or community culture that has patriarchal social structures, but is not unknown in more individualist Western culture.[7] Whilst the traditional forms of FGM have all but disappeared in the West – except, covertly, within immigrant communities – it continues in the developing world.

In the UK and USA, there is evidence that in the nineteenth century the practice of FGM was performed by gynaecologists to cure so-called female weaknesses – nymphomania, insanity, masturbation and other 'female disorders', for example – and now transcends and crosses all religious, racial and social boundaries.[8]

Prevalence of FGM

Due to lack of systematic data collection, precise numbers of women and girls who have undergone FGM is unknown, but it is estimated that 120–140 million women and girls worldwide will have undergone the traditional practice of FGM in some form or another and millions more are at risk.[9] Prevalence is still high in around 28–30 countries in Africa and the Middle East[10] and can also be traced to

Table 1.1 The prevalence of FGM[13]

Country	Prevalence (%)	Year
Benin	50	1996
Burkina Faso	72	1999
Cameroon	20	1998
Central African Republic	43	1994
Chad	60	1996/97
Côte d'Ivoire	43	1994
Dem. Rep. of Congo (formerly Zaire)	5	Unknown
Djibouti	98	Unknown
Egypt	97	1995
Eritrea	95	1995
Ethiopia	85	1984/1990
Gambia	80	1985
Ghana	80	1998
Guinea	99	1999
Guinea-Bissau	50	1990
Kenya	38	1998
Liberia	60	1986
Mali	94	1996
Mauritania	25	1987
Niger	5	1998
Nigeria	40–50	Various years
Senegal	20	1999
Sierra Leone	90	1987
Somalia	98–100	1982–1993
Sudan	89	1990
Tanzania	18	1996
Togo	12	1996
Uganda	5	1995/6
Yemen	23	1997

Latin America, India, Malaysia and Indonesia (see Table 1.1). Its incidence is estimated to range from 50% to 98%.[11,12]

This would be an appropriate time to address the issue of terminology. The World Health Organization (WHO), UNICEF, and many of those opposed to the practice of FGM use the term 'female genital mutilation', but others adopt variations, for example, 'female circumcision', 'female genital alteration', 'female genital cutting' and 'female genital excision'.

FGM encompasses all procedures involving partial or total removal of the external female genitalia or other injury to the female genital organs, whether for cultural, religious or other non-therapeutic reasons. There are different types of FGM; they include:

- **Type 1:** Excision of the prepuce, with or without excision of part or all of the clitoris.
- **Type 2:** Excision of the clitoris with partial or total excision of the labia minora.
- **Type 3:** Excision of part or all of the external genitalia and stitching/narrowing of the vaginal opening (infibulation).

- **Type 4:** Pricking, piercing or incising of the clitoris and/or labia; stretching of the clitoris and/or labia; cauterisation by burning of the clitoris and surrounding tissue. Scraping of tissue surrounding the vaginal orifice (angurya cuts) or cutting of the vagina (gishiri cuts). Introduction of corrosive substances or herbs into the vagina to cause bleeding or for the purpose of tightening or narrowing it, and any other procedure that falls under the definition given above[9] (*see* Figure 1.1).

FGM procedures

The procedures described above are irreversible and last a lifetime.[10] In urban areas, FGM is now more frequently performed in hospitals, by trained doctors and midwives, with sterile equipment and use of general or local anaesthesia to reduce pain.[6,14] However, carrying out the procedure in hospital does not make any difference to the risk of short- and long-term complications; it violates the Hippocratic Oath's credo 'to do no harm' and is unethical by any standards.[2,13]

Elsewhere, anaesthetic and antiseptics are not widely used and the procedure may be carried out using crude tools and instruments: razors, knives and scissors (*see* 1, colour plate section).

In Type 3 excision or infibulation (*see* Figure 1.1), elderly women, relatives and friends secure the girl in the lithotomy position. A deep incision is made rapidly on either side from the root of the clitoris to the fourchette, and a single cut of the razor excises the clitoris and both the labia majora and the labia minora.

Bleeding is profuse, but is usually controlled by the application of various poultices, the threading of the edges of the skin with thorns, or clasping them between the edges of a split cane. A piece of twig is inserted between the edges of the skin to ensure a patent foramen for urinary and menstrual flow. The lower limbs are then bound together for 2–6 weeks to promote haemostasis and encourage union of the two sides (*see* 2, colour plate section).[15]

Healing takes place by primary intention, and, as a result, the introitus is obliterated by a drum of skin extending across the orifice except for a small hole.[14,16,17] Circumstances at the time may vary; the girl may struggle ferociously, in which case the incisions may become uncontrolled and haphazard. The girl may be pinned down so firmly that bones may fracture.

Consequences of FGM

FGM poses considerable health risks, exacerbated by the procedure often being performed in unhygienic conditions by untrained individuals. There is widespread concern amongst international organisations about the potentially fatal short-term and long-term consequences of FGM, multiple use of 'instruments' in transmission of HIV and the potentially devastating physical and psychosexual effects of FGM.[18]

Health complications of FGM have been described as the 'three feminine sorrows' (*see* below). Sorrows on the day FGM takes place, the night of the wedding where often the woman has to be cut prior to intercourse and when the woman gives birth and the vaginal opening is not large enough for a safe delivery.[19]

For approximately 10% of girls and women, the short-term complications of FGM – haemorrhage, shock and infection, for example – have fatal consequences.

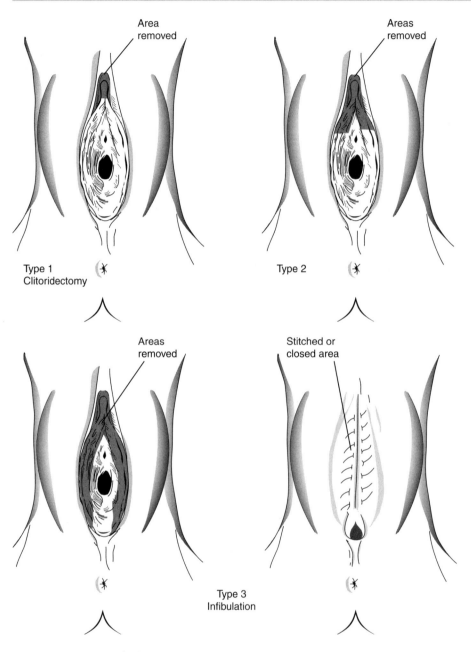

Figure 1.1 Types of FGM

A further 25% die in the long term, as a result of recurrent urinary and vaginal infections and complications during childbirth, such as severe bleeding and obstructed labour. Complications can be separated into the immediate and later complications.

Immediate complications, as reported by some 39% of women in Somalia, include haemorrhage, infection, tetanus and trauma to adjacent tissues, septicaemia, shock and death. Long-term complications include impaired urinary and menstrual function, vaginal stenosis, chronic genital pain (from pelvic inflammatory disease), cysts, neuromas, ulcers, infertility and incontinence from vesico-vaginal fistula (VVF). Psychosocial and psychosexual consequences can also present. Childbirth requires cutting and repairing the infibulation, which causes additional morbidity and increases the chances of maternal and child mortality, though this does not occur in the West.

Three feminine sorrows

And if I may speak of my wedding night:
I had expected caresses. Sweet kisses. Hugging and love.
No. Never.
Awaiting me was pain. Suffering and sadness.
I lay in my wedding bed, groaning like a wounded animal, a victim of feminine pain.
At dawn, ridicule awaited me. My mother announced: Yes she is a virgin.
When fear gets hold of me. When anger seizes my body.
When hate becomes my companion, then I get feminine advice, because it is only feminine pain.
And I am told feminine pain perishes like all feminine things.
The journey continues. Or the struggle continues.
As modern historians say, as the good tie of marriage matures.
As I submit and sorrow subsides, my belly becomes like a balloon.
A glimpse of happiness shows, a hope. A new baby. A new life!
But a new life endangers my life.
A baby's birth is death and destruction for me!
It is what my grandmother called the three feminine sorrows.
She said the day of circumcision; the wedding night and the birth of a baby are the triple feminine sorrows.
As the birth bursts, I cry for help, when the battered flesh tears.
No mercy. Push! They say. It is only feminine pain!
And now I appeal: I appeal for love lost, for dreams broken, for the right to live as a whole human being.
I appeal to all peace loving people to protect, to support and give a hand to innocent little girls who do no harm.
Obedient to their parents and elders, all they know is only smiles.
Initiate them to the world of love, not the world of feminine sorrows.
Poem by a woman of courage in Somalia
(Her name has been withheld to protect her anonymity)

Why FGM continues

It is useful to explore the rationale of those who perpetuate the practice of FGM in these so-called enlightened times. The most common reason is tradition, but the other main components are psychosexual, religious, sociological and for hygienic and aesthetic purposes (*see* Figure 1.2).[20]

Many of the reasons offered for performing FGM have been dispelled as myth or medically discredited. However, to understand why the above-mentioned traditional beliefs still persist in parts of Africa, the Middle East and Asia, one has to revisit the history of FGM and examine the social structures that have been, and continue to be, in place in areas where FGM remains prevalent.

Older women in these communities perceive continuance of FGM as preserving the very fabric of their society. For women in such societies, marriage equates with security and stability. As a married woman who has reached maturity, she now has the ability to satisfy the needs of her husband and can be assured of a secure and stable life. By contrast, failure to have a daughter circumcised is tantamount to condemning her to social isolation and disgrace for her family.[21,22]

Employment opportunities for women in such societies are limited and performing FGM is, in many cases, their only source of revenue. Work is being done to educate women about how they might replace this income with other types of work, but convincing them to discuss issues of female genitalia, women's sexuality

---

Psychosexual

- A woman's virginity is an absolute prerequisite for marriage.
- In Egypt and Sudan, female circumcision is seen to increase male sexual pleasure during intercourse.
- The clitoris is seen as an aggressive organ that threatens the male penis.
- Presence of the clitoris endangers baby during delivery.
- Alternatively, the clitoris is seen as central to sexual desire and its excision protects a woman from her over-sexed nature and saves her from temptation and disgrace whilst preserving her virtue.

Religious

- Clitoridectomy is believed to have its origins in African institutions and to have been adopted by Islam at the conquest of Egypt in 742 AD.

Note: Female circumcision transcends religious boundaries and female circumcision is not practised in most Islamic countries and is not in accordance with the Koran.

Social

- An initiation rite of development into adulthood, becoming a mature woman.
- Socialisation of female fertility.
- The ceremonial that often surrounds female circumcision is intended to teach young girls about her duties as a wife and mother.

Aesthetic

- In some societies the clitoris is considered unpleasant and ugly to sight and touch.
- Removal of the 'unsightly' female genitalia is deemed a sign of maturity.
- Female circumcision maintains the women's physical and mental health.

Figure 1.2 Elements of rationale for practice of FGM

and FGM is complex. Westerners working to eradicate FGM are often viewed with suspicion, seeking to impose their Western ways upon people. However, activists are increasingly from Africa, the Middle East and Asia.

On a recent visit to Somalia (*see 3*, colour plate section), it was possible to gain some awareness of present attitudes to FGM, where people not trained in surgery (parents, grandparents and traditional birth attendants) largely perform FGM. Before the collapse of the Somali government in 1991, there was support for the eradication of female circumcision. The practice was banished from hospitals and health research was conducted. A decade of civil war, however, put a stop to any attempts at co-ordinated national action and today, according to the WHO, Somalia has one of the highest rates of female circumcision of any country (98%); the most extreme form, Pharaonic/infibulation, is the most widely practised.

Somaliland was chosen to visit because almost 90% of women/girls seen at my clinic are from Somalia. The practice of female circumcision has continued to thrive in Somalia despite traditional birth attendants' recognition of its complications, because of strongly held cultural and religious beliefs. Traditional birth attendants, willing in theory to curtail the practice, continue to do so because most parents persist in demanding it. Parents more aware of health issues do not have their daughters infibulated but they remain in the minority. A large proportion of the population favour female circumcision despite vivid childhood memories of many Somali women.

It is important to understand that, in the context of promoting change of attitudes to the practice of FGM, change agents must use language that is acceptable to the target group if they are to avoid polarising the very people they want to reach. Failure to do this will undoubtedly lead to misunderstanding, misinterpretation and a perception amongst African and Arab cultures in particular of Westerners devaluing their culture.[23,24]

References

1   El Dareer A (1983) Epidemiology of female circumcision in the Sudan. *Trop Doct*. **13**: 41–5.
2   Eke N (2000) Female genital mutilation: what can be done? *Lancet*. **356**(Supplement): 57.
3   Izett S and Toubia N (1999) *A Research and Evaluation Guidebook Using Female Circumcision as a Case Study: Learning about social changes*. Rainbo, New York.
4   Wasunna A (2000) Towards redirecting the female circumcision debate: legal, ethical and cultural considerations. *MJM*. **5**: 104–10.
5   Barnes-Dean V (1985) Clitoridectomy and infibulation. *Cultural Survival Quarterly*. **9.2**: 1–8.
6   Bridgehouse R (1992) Ritual female circumcision and its effects on female sexual function. *Can J Hum Sexuality*. **1**: 3–10.
7   Hellsten SK (2004) Rationalising circumcision: from tradition to fashion, from public health to individual freedom – critical notes on cultural persistence of the practice of genital mutilation. *Med Ethics*. **30**: 248–53.
8   Webb E (1995) Female genital mutilation. Cultural knowledge is the key to understanding. *BMJ*. **70**: 441–4.
9   World Health Organization (2000) *Factsheet 241*. World Health Organization, Geneva.
10 World Health Organization (1997) *FGM: a joint WHO/UNICEF/UNFPA statement*. World Health Organization, Geneva.
11 Dorkenoo E (1995) *Cutting the Rose: female genital mutilation: the practice and its prevention*. Minority Rights Publications, London.

12 Toubia N (1999) *A Technical Manual for Health Care Providers Caring for Women With Circumcision.* Rainbo, New York.

13 World Health Organization (2001) *A Teacher's Guide: integrating the prevention and management of the health complication into the curricula of nursing and midwifery.* World Health Organization, Geneva.

14 McCaffery M (1995) Management of female genital mutilation. Northwick Park Hospital experience. *Br J Obstet Gynaecol.* **102**: 787–90.

15 World Health Organization (1996) *Female Genital Mutilation: a report of the WHO Technical Working Group.* World Health Organization, Geneva.

16 Momoh C (1999) Female genital mutilation: the struggle continues. *Pract Nurs.* **10**: 31–3.

17 Toubia N (1999) *A Technical Manual for Health Care Providers Caring for Women With Circumcision.* Rainbo, New York.

18 UNYANZ National Model United Nations/WHO (2004) *Question of eradication of female genital mutilation.* UNYANZ, Geneva.

19 Fourcroy JL (1998) The three feminine sorrows. *Hospital Practice.* **33**: 15–21

20 Epelboin S and Epelboin A (1979) Special report: female circumcision. *People.* **6**: 24–9.

21 Lightfoot-Klein H (1989) *Prisoners of Ritual: an odyssey into female genital mutilation in Africa.* Haworth Press, New York.

22 Hosken FP (1993) *The Hosken Report: genital and sexual mutilation of females.* Women's International Network News, Lexington MA.

23 Davis DS (2001) Male and female genital alteration: a collision course with the law? *Journal of Law-Medicine.* **11**: 487–570.

24 National Women's Health Information Center (NWHIC 2001) *Female Genital Cutting: frequently asked questions.* NWHIC, Project of US Department of Health and Human Services.

Chapter Two

FGM and issues of gender and human rights of women

Comfort Momoh

Introduction

Perpetuation of the practice of FGM cannot be fully understood without exploring the issues of gender and women's human rights. 'Gender' is a term given to the social construction of roles allocated to men and women,[1] and shouldn't be confused with 'sex', which we are born into; women menstruate, are able to become pregnant, give birth and breastfeed an infant, for example. Men can produce and impregnate women with sperm,[2] but, at the risk of stating the obvious, what the two sexes cannot do is swap these functions.

Gender, on the other hand – how we act within our socio-cultural roles, as men and women – can change over time, due in part to societies' expectations and constraints placed upon men and women by virtue of their sex.[3] Indeed, psychologists and sociologists argue that gender roles are assigned at birth. Northern, for example, maintains that, as soon as people put a label 'girl' or 'boy' on the child, they begin treating that child in a stereotypical fashion.[4]

Knowledge of gender affords us the opportunity to increase our understanding of how and why men and women act (behave) in the way they do. An insight into the differing roles men and women play in society and the rights and responsibilities that come with these roles is essential to building effective working relationships with men and women.

Gender roles are based on stereotypes[5] and the family, school, peers, work supervisors and the mass media, for example, then reinforce 'conventions' throughout the lifespan.[5] Let us consider for a moment how each of us might, at some time, have put a label on someone. What did you last buy for your daughter's birthday? Who is more likely to help Dad repair the car, son or daughter? Which sex is under-represented in the professions? Which is perceived as 'the gentle sex' and who holds the power and or controls a relationship?

'Power' is a broad concept; in the context of continuance of the practice of FGM, it relates to men having power over women in making decisions about all aspects of girls'/women's role in society, local community's expectations, intimate personal relationships, and family planning and childbearing. The extent of power imbalance will depend on men and women's culture, socio-economic pressures, level of education and access to media, employment opportunities and the resources at their disposal to do with as they please.[6]

Many women living in communities that practise FGM have few if any personal expectations for the future, perceiving their life map as being predictable and determined by those in positions of control. Sexual intercourse continues to be defined in terms of women satisfying the needs and desires of the dominant male and women will often find it impossible to articulate their own needs, either because they don't know how to or for fear of rejection, domestic violence and or abandonment and subsequent loss of social and financial security.

Kohlberg believed that children should acquire awareness and understanding of gender before socialisation influences them; at three years old, a child knows what sex they are. At between five and seven years, they can appreciate that their 'boy' or 'girl' label will not change. Later, children come to realise that boys become men and girls become women.[7]

Social learning theorists explained gender stereotyping of occupations; parents and teachers 'encourage' each sex to pursue academic subjects and/or careers that are deemed 'gender-appropriate'. This is illustrated by children who aspire to occupations that fit their own gender; children imitate, watching the work that adults of the same sex as them pursue. They also quickly pick up gender traits and expectations of certain gender-related actions.[7]

In Western cultures disparities have become somewhat blurred but, in East Africa for example, gender differences are clear. Largely speaking, women have no power or influence; they have little access to education and are totally dominated by men. Despite their significant contribution to daily survival, they have no money of their own to spend as they wish and are often subject to domestic violence, exploitation and abuse.[4]

Violence against women is an age-old problem that can be found in every culture and social group.[8] In 1993 the United Nations (UN) defined such violence in the Declaration on the Elimination of Violence Against Women. Article 1 stated that violence against women includes,

> Any act of gender-based violence that results in, or is likely to result in, physical, sexual or psychological harm or suffering to women, including threats of such acts, coercion or arbitrary deprivations of liberty, whether occurring in public or private life.[9]

For families who come to the West, as refugees or asylum seekers, the notion of the male head of household helping out with the chores or adopting a role in the upbringing of their children, particularly during infancy, is incomprehensible and the mothers of sons reinforce such traditional concepts, not expecting or even daring to suggest that it is okay for their sons to babysit their female sibling, wash up or do some shopping, for instance.

Fundamental to the welfare of the child is to be brought up in a family unit where both the mother and father are involved in the nurturing and support of their children in an atmosphere where relations between men and women in that family are based on equal rights and shared responsibilities. For this to become a reality, in particular, in patriarchal societies, organisations like UNICEF are targeting and including men in discussions and education strategies that facilitate adaptation of roles within the family. If men can be sold the idea that being a role model to children should be based on mutual respect and equitable opportunities for men and women, it is anticipated that women will benefit in terms of decreased domestic violence and sexual exploitation, and men taking a different gender perspective.[10]

Human rights of women

Violence against women is an important but often hidden issue in the West, FGM being one example. In 1995 Amnesty International (AI) decided to include the issue of FGM in its promotional work on human rights. In doing so, AI recognised the urgency of taking a position against this widespread form of violence against women prior to the Fourth UN World Conference on Women held in Beijing in September 1995.[11] In March 2004 AI launched a worldwide campaign to eradicate violence against women.

The traditional practice of FGM is perceived as necessary if a girl is to become a complete woman and is a clear example of a practice that 'marks the divergence of the sexes in terms of their future roles in life and marriage'.[11] In many countries, where emphasis is placed on customs, rituals and tradition, violence against women in this context is either condoned or accepted as a way of life. FGM is one example of this form of violence; such cases of brutality only occur against women and are motivated either by their sex or their social roles in society.[12]

It was many years before FGM was regarded as a human rights issue; such practices were viewed as a 'private matter'. But human rights implications are now recognised at international level. FGM is representative of oppression of women that has its foundation in manipulation of women's sexuality, intended to maintain male dominance and exploitation. This is based on an ideology amongst societies that perpetuate the practice that women should be 'shaped and moulded, cut and tucked into a more appealing commodity for man's pleasures'.[13]

FGM is a violation of women's physical and psychological integrity and an impediment to health and well-being that has challenged activists worldwide. Despite public condemnation and pressure on governments to end this deeply entrenched practice, it still persists. One illustration is that although FGM is largely performed on girls (9–19 years of age), in Kenya FGM has been known to be forcefully undertaken on women as old as 60 years of age.[14]

In December 2001, Kenya's President Moi issued a decree against FGM but in the absence of legislation specific to FGM, action can only be taken under provisions of the Penal Code relating to assault and bodily harm. Dr Okumu argues that formal and informal education about FGM is required and medical practitioners should be trained to manage cases of FGM. He also maintains that the Penal Code must be amended to specifically address FGM.[14]

The Director-General of the World Health Organization believes it wholly unacceptable that,

> The international community remain passive in the name of a distorted vision of multiculturalism ... People will change their behaviour when they understand the hazards and indignity of harmful practices and when they realise that it is possible to give up harmful practices without giving up meaningful aspects of their culture.[15]

Dorkenoo contends that,

> To succeed in abolishing the practice of FGM will demand fundamental attitudinal shifts in the way that society perceives the human rights of women.[16]

There are a number of principles already in place that point towards an obligation on governments to take appropriate and effective action. The Universal Declaration of Human Rights (UDHR 1948) is recognised as a common standard that aims to promote respect for the rights and freedoms of all human beings and demands that they should 'act towards one another in a spirit of brotherhood'. It makes abundantly clear that all have the right not to be subjected to cruel, inhuman or degrading treatment, which is of direct relevance to FGM.*

Whilst embracing the basic concept of human rights enshrined in the Declaration, many governments have failed to apply them to abuses within the home or community. The UN Convention on the Elimination of All Forms of Discrimination against Women (CEDAW 1981) has, to 2004, 176 signatories and is often described as a bill of rights for women.[†] This makes explicit reference to traditional practices that are based on the idea of 'inferiority or superiority of either of the sexes', infringing their human rights and integrity.

The Convention is monitored by the Committee on CEDAW, which recommends that states must adopt appropriate effective action to prevent, punish and eradicate, for example, FGM through healthcare, advice and education.[‡] The UN Declaration on the Elimination of Violence against Women (1993) refers specifically to gender-based violence 'both in public or private life'. This principle was reaffirmed at the Fourth UN World Conference on Women held in Beijing in September 1995.

Working to empower women

International, national and regional conferences have recognised as fundamental to global development the importance of women being able to gain greater equality with men. In the West, most women enjoy greater self-esteem and control over their own lives and men should take some of the credit for this situation, having accepted their changing roles in society. Many governments of African nations, too, have taken measures to give women socio-economic and political rights. Men and women are working worldwide to educate communities by holding support groups, conducting seminars and training sessions; governments are introducing or tightening up legislation outlawing the practice of FGM; there is expanding research on women's issues; and community and religious leaders are using their influence to facilitate public declarations to stop the practice.

In Eritrea, for example, the Constitution prohibits discrimination against women, children and the disabled, and these are enforced. It was recognised that

---

* On 10 December 10 1948 the General Assembly of the United Nations adopted and proclaimed the Universal Declaration of Human Rights. Following this historic act the Assembly called upon all member countries to publicise the text of the Declaration and 'to cause it to be disseminated, displayed, read and expounded principally in schools and other educational institutions, without distinction based on the political status of countries or territories'.

[†] The Convention on the Elimination of All Forms of Discrimination against Women (CEDAW), adopted in 1979 by the UN General Assembly, consists of a preamble and 30 articles. It defines what constitutes discrimination against women and sets up an agenda for national action to end such discrimination.

[‡] The United Nations Committee on the Elimination of Discrimination against Women (CEDAW), an expert body established in 1982, is composed of 23 experts on women's issues from around the world.

women played a significant role, as fighters, in the struggle for independence and since Eritrea's independence women have enjoyed a legal right to equal educational opportunities, equal pay for equal work and legal sanctions against domestic violence.

The East African Media Women's Association (EAMWA) acknowledges that Eritrea's government has recognised women's role in society, evidenced by the fact that there are a number of women occupying high government posts, with 22% of the members of parliament, 11.1% of the ambassadors and 16% of the judges being women.* However, there are some disparities, mainly in rural communities, where much of society remains traditional and patriarchal, there are ingrained cultural attitudes and most women have an inferior status to men in their homes and communities. FGM is undergone by 95% of females in Eritrea and there is no law prohibiting FGM, though the government does discourage the practice.

Organisations like Black Women's Health and Family Support and Womankind Worldwide, for example, develop practical programmes in partnership with local, regional and national groups to tackle women's inequality in many of the world's poorest places. Those projects work to unlock women's potential and maximise their ability to make decisions about their own lives and the lives of their families, as well as contribute to the future of their community and country. They challenge the unacceptable level of gender inequality.

Simply making FGM illegal and punishing those who carry out the practice is not enough, since it is inextricably bound up with livelihoods, community identification and women's status, and therefore a more holistic approach is taken. Association of African Women for Research and Development (AAWORD) firmly condemns FGM as a serious violation of the fundamental rights of women. They argue, however, that,

> In order to be effective, westerners should attempt to fight against FGM by placing it in the context of ignorance and poverty and by questioning the structures and social relations that perpetuate the situation.[17]

In Mali, 91.6% of all women aged 15–49 years have undergone FGM. Among all adult women, 92.5% were mutilated. The children's charity Plan International is running a five-year campaign in Mali to raise awareness of the harm caused by FGM and aims to spread the message via radio, traditional songs, women's groups and Muslim religious leaders. Mali is a staunchly Islamic country but Plan International is trying hard to spread the message that there is nothing in the Koran or other Islamic religious texts that calls for this procedure to be performed.[†]

Amongst Mauritania's minority peoples, especially in the South, almost every girl is subjected to the ritual of FGM. The Mauritanian government generally has a relatively good record on promoting women's rights, but eradication of FGM is not seen as a priority. On the contrary, the government representatives have tried to justify these practices before the Committee in the name of cultural relativism

---

* East African Media Women's Association (EAMWA) launched a website on 8 March 2001. EAMWA attempts to empower women journalists through professional education and training.
† Plan International helps create lasting improvements to the lives of children, their families and communities in over 40 developing countries. PLAN's belief is in working together with communities to identify their needs and meet them in the most appropriate, long-term and sustainable ways.

but Committee on the Elimination of Racial Discrimination (CERD) has urged the government to 'put an end to these practices'.[18]

In Kenya, FGM is most prevalent in the northeast of the country, with an estimated 98% of girls aged 5–9 years undergoing infibulation, citing FGM as a requirement of the Islamic faith. MAYO and PATH are establishing alternative ceremonials to celebrate rites of passage into womanhood. In communities where FGM is traditionally carried out on girls at puberty, the alternative involves taking the girls into seclusion to train to be future wives and mothers, leaving out the actual cut, but there has been resistance where the practice is entrenched.[19]

To address this challenge, moves are being undertaken to work with Kenya's Ministry of Education to include anti-FGM messages in school curriculum.* Anti-FGM campaigners are also having to address so-called 'sanitised practice', which involves medical professionals illegally performing FGM.[16] Although FGM is outlawed in Kenya under the Children's Act (2002), the ambiguities in the Act have left the judiciary uncertain as to appropriate punishment to impose on offenders.

There is no doubt that views are changing regarding FGM. In countries like Egypt, Somalia and Ethiopia, more than 90% have been circumcised but numbers are decreasing; in Egypt, for example, FGM has been reduced from 96% to approximately 84% of the total female population. UNICEF began anti-FGM programmes in Egypt in 1998, educating parents of the dangers of FGM, but it acknowledges that eradication of FGM will take time despite changing attitudes. UNICEF[†] argues that governments must abide by commitments they made at the UN Special Session on Children and move immediately to end the disturbing phenomenon by 2010.[20]

African governments are facing increasing demands to toughen laws to stamp out FGM. Only 16 African countries, including Ethiopia, have adopted laws to protect women and girls from the ancient custom, which is also blamed for spreading HIV/AIDS. The Inter-African Committee on Traditional Practices (IAC) collaborated with the Organisation of African Unity (OAU) to prepare a protocol for elimination of harmful practices which are contrary to international standards.[21] But at a conference to mark the international day of Zero Tolerance to FGM, the President of IAC said more action needed to be taken because, despite the introduction of legislation, the laws were not always enforced.[22]

Somali culture is patriarchal but the situation of urban women is undergoing change, with women exercising their democratic and political rights (see 4, colour plate section).

That said, men do still hold the balance of power in the country; in the rural areas, the roles of women have changed very little and traditional culture and beliefs remain embedded in the community's psyche. WOMANKIND reports that a 1999 CARE International survey estimates 100% prevalence in Somaliland, the overwhelming majority being Type 3 infibulation.[23]

Steps have been taken to explore how Europe and Africa can work together to ban FGM as, due to migration and refugee movements, the issue has become one of global concern that must be dealt with on an international scale. Despite

---

* Equality Now, a New York-based international NGO campaigning for women's rights, convened a meeting in Nairobi, which brought together former FGM practitioners.
† UNICEF is committed to eliminating all forms of FGM. The organisation's work focuses on building a protective environment for children that safeguards them from abuse and exploitation.

legislation put in place by many European nations, prosecutions are few, and Europe must be committed to widespread condemnation of the practice. No nation can bury their head in the sand; FORWARD, a UK rights group, estimates that there are still significant numbers of new cases every year in the UK and many of these women and girls do not know where to seek advice and medical assistance.*

In concluding this chapter, it is important for the reader to appreciate that there is only scope here to provide a snapshot of the issue of gender as it relates to women's right to physical and psychological integrity, empowerment and features associated with the practice of FGM. Whilst examples have been given of work being done by NGOs to raise awareness of FGM as a breach of human rights, it has been impossible to acknowledge all the people worldwide – religious leaders, men (*see* 5, colour plate section) and women (*see* 6, colour plate section) – who are meeting the challenge and taking steps towards eradicating FGM, most especially those who have had the courage to confront their community, perceived cultural norms and inherent values and beliefs. This, however, does not in any way diminish their efforts and you are urged to access the literature available for further information.

References

1   O'Brien O and White A (2003) *Gender and Health: The case for gender-sensitive health policy and health care delivery.* Conference Paper for 14 November 2003. King's Fund, London.
2   Green M (2000) *Newsletter: Gender and Health Promotion.* Centre for Health Promotion Research, Leeds Metropolitan University, Leeds.
3   Gijsbers Van Wijk CM, Van Vliet KP and Kolk AM (1996) Gender perspectives and quality of care: towards appropriate and adequate health care for women. *Social Science and Medicine.* **43**(5): 707–20.
4   Northern D *Gender Issues.* St. Augustine University of Tanzania. Electronic Publications, Tanzania.
5   Kean M-L (1995) *Gender Roles, Gender Identity and Sexual Orientation.* Psychology 9A Lecture 19 Notes.
6   Raghavan-Gilbert VW (1999) *Gender.* PowerPoint Presentation, UNFPA: Country support team for the South Pacific.
7   Helwig AA (1998) Gender-role stereotyping: testing theory with a longitudinal sample. *Sex Roles: A Journal of Research.* **March.** 403–23.
8   UNIFEM (2001) *Factsheet No 5: Masculinity and Gender Violence.* UNIFEM.
9   United Nations (1993) *Declaration on the Elimination of Violence Against Women. Article 1.* UN, New York.
10 Foumbi J and Lovich R (1997) *Role of Men in the Lives of Children: a study on how improving knowledge about men in families helps strengthen programming for children and women.* NYHQ: UNICEF.
11 UNICEF (2003) *Female Genital Mutilation: Sections 1 & 2.* UNICEF.
12 SADC (1998) *Conference Notes: Prevention of Violence Against Women: Summary Report.* SADC, 5–8 March.
13 Get Ethical (2003) *Female Genital Mutilation.* Juretic Media Ltd. http://www.ethicalmatters.co.uk
14 Dorkenoo E (1995) *Cutting the Rose. Female genital mutilation: the practice and its prevention.* Minority Rights Publications, London.

---

*FORWARD is concerned with empowering women in the hope that this will end the practice of FGM.

15 Okumu C Dr (2002) Right to bodily and psychological integrity: are reproductive rights a constitutional issue? In: A Ghirmazion, A Nyabera and E Wanjugu Kamweru (eds) *Perspectives on Global Discourse: gender and constitution-making in Kenya*. Heinrich Böll Foundation, East and Horn of Africa.

16 Statement of the Director-General to the World Health Organization's Global Commission on Women's Health, 12 April 1994.

17 Hermon-Kiernan H (2003) *FGM: Ethical Matters*. Get Ethical. WOMANKIND, London.

18 Committee on the Elimination of Racial Discrimination (CERD) Session (Geneva, 2 to 20 August 2004).

19 Kenya National Focal Point for FGM. In: UN Office for the Coordination of Humanitarian Affairs, Friday 11 June 2004.

20 UNICEF (2003) *UNICEF calls on governments to fulfil pledge to end female genital mutilation*. UNICEF, New York.

21 Inter-African Committee (IAC 2000) *Newsletter No. 28, December*. IAC.

22 Ras-Work B (2004) *Conference Delegates in Ethiopia Call for End to FGM*. Addis Ababa, Ethiopia.

23 WOMANKIND (2003) *Womankind's Work in Somalia*. WOMANKIND, London.

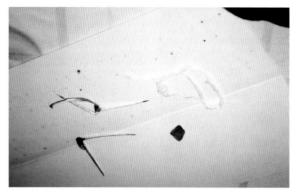

1. Equipment for circumcision

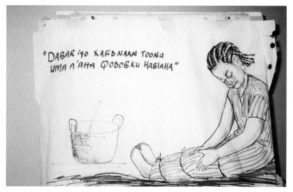

2. A wall hanging in Somalia

Plates 1-6 taken in Somalia by Comfort Momoh

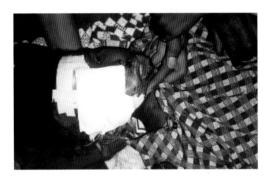

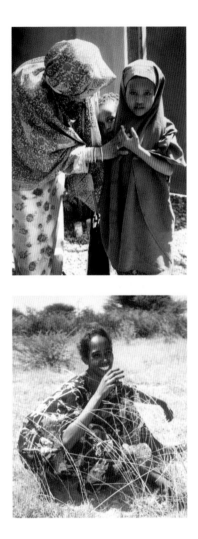

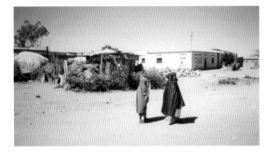

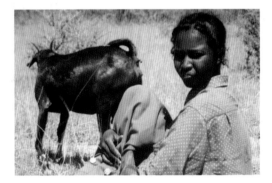

3. These pictures give a flavour of life as lived by the people of Somalia; it must not be assumed that the women and girls depicted have all undergone FGM

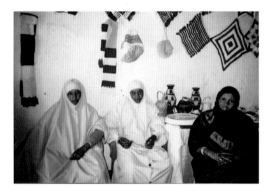

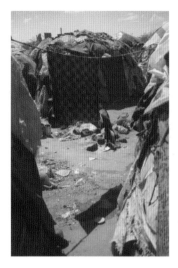

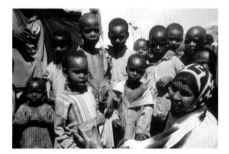

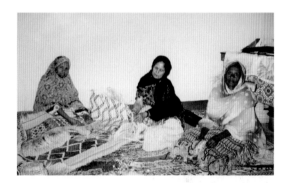

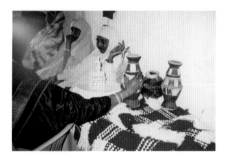

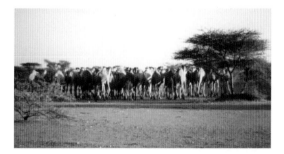

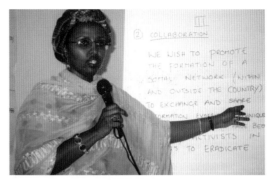

4. Women moving towards empowerment

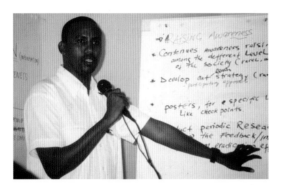

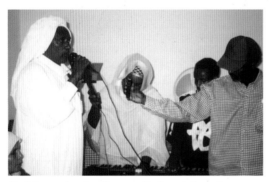

5. Men, including religious leaders, are beginning to mobilise

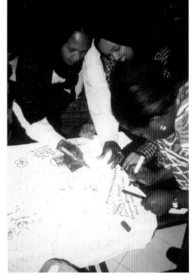

6. Women signing a cloth to support the campaign to end FGM globally

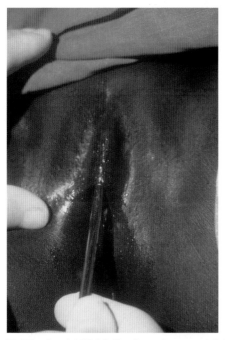

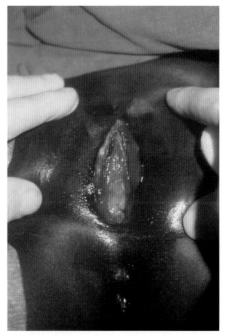

7. Typical FGM 3 showing a thick layer of scar tissue across the introitus

8. De-fibulation of the case shown in picture 7; the clitoris and hood of the clitoris are clearly seen

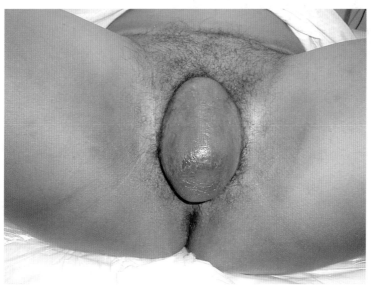

9. Demoid cyst – one of the complications of FGM

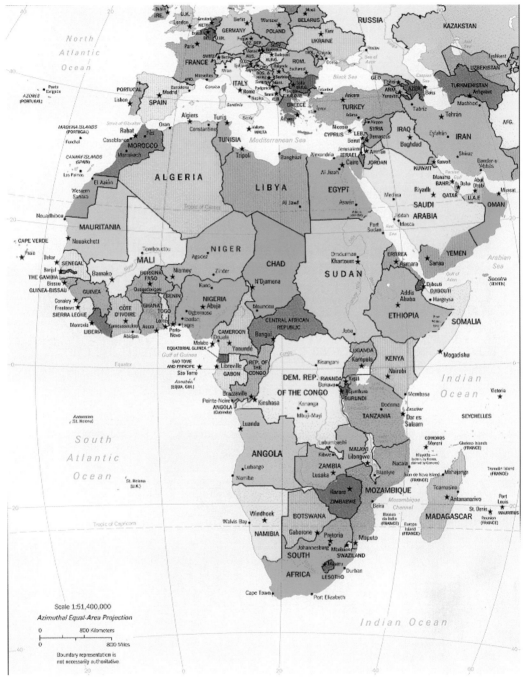

10. Map of Africa

Chapter Three

Managing the reality of FGM in the UK

Janice Rymer and Comfort Momoh

Background

Women with female genital mutilation (FGM) have very specific medical, gynaecological, obstetric and psychological problems, which doctors and midwives are not usually trained to treat.[1–4] The covert nature of this ritualistic practice and illegality of the procedure has meant that there are few opportunities for those working in the field of obstetrics and gynaecology to build knowledge, skills and experience of dealing with this client group.[5]

The practice of FGM is centuries old. It is often described as a tribal practice; however, clitoridectomy was performed on women in England until the nineteenth century, amidst fears of female promiscuity and 'sexually deviant' habits like masturbation. Such perceptions of the need for FGM were later discredited and later came increased female emancipation and the emergence of the sexual revolution of the 'swinging 60s'.

During the 1980s FGM resurfaced with the arrival of immigrants, students, refugees and asylum seekers from countries that had continued FGM on their daughters, for example, Somalia, Ethiopia, Djibouti, Sudan and Eritrea.[6] Health professionals were undoubtedly ill-prepared for managing the care and treatment of these women and this was compounded by the fact that there was little or no understanding of the multiplicity of gender-related socio-cultural and economic factors underpinning FGM.

There is a great deal of evidence to suggest that female asylum seekers face particular difficulties, which are often unacknowledged.[7] These women frequently have little or no knowledge of gynaecological and obstetric services available to them and often do not speak sufficient English to be able to access advice and support. This is where organisations like Black Women's Health and Family Support (BWHFS) are invaluable in providing a link between such women and healthcare professionals who need to be sensitive to their background, culture and experiences.

They should be offered a choice as to the gender of healthcare professionals and interpreters and be encouraged to access screening and health promotion programmes. As they often feel lonely and isolated, they may welcome the opportunity to belong to a group and, once again, non-governmental organisations and charitable organisations can assist in putting women in contact with other women who share their culture.[7] This is particularly helpful to women who have undergone FGM and mothers of female children who are now living, temporarily or permanently, in the UK. While there may be nurses, midwives, health visitors, social workers and clinicians who might never come across women and girls with FGM during their professional lives, the possibility is increasing for the reasons mentioned above, and they must be prepared with the necessary knowledge and skills and the right attitude to manage care and treatment appropriately and be able to supply information and advice regarding the dangers of FGM as well as making families aware that FGM is unacceptable and illegal in the UK and parents are not permitted to take female children abroad for 'holidays' for the purpose of FGM.[8]

There are 74 000 African immigrant women living in the UK who have undergone some form of FGM and 7000 under-16-year-olds who are thought to be at risk. Damage to the anatomy caused by the procedure is irreversible.[7] Women with FGM may present late into a pregnancy and those who have been infibulated (the woman's vagina is stitched, leaving a very narrow opening and her external genitalia, including the clitoris, are removed) will need a reversal before they can give birth. This involves opening up the vagina so that the baby can be delivered. Some women actively choose to wait to have reversal until they go into labour; they dread the prospect of reliving the prepubescent childhood experience of FGM and often suffer flashbacks to the original mutilation.[9]

Presenting complications

Female genital mutilation (FGM) is removal of part or all of the female external genitalia (*see* Chapter 2). It ranges from being very simple to the radical form, and is usually carried out sometime between birth and puberty. The medical complications can be divided as follows:

1 immediate complications
2 intermediate complications
3 long-term complications
4 sexual dysfunction
5 problems with inadequate gynaecological examination
6 early pregnancy problems
7 problems in labour
8 post-partum problems
9 psychological sequelae.

Immediate complications

A traditional practitioner who has had no surgical training usually performs the procedure itself. The environment is usually far removed from an operating theatre and there is usually minimal attempt to ensure a sterile procedure. The instruments used may be knives, razor blades or glass. No anaesthetic is used and relatives and or friends usually hold down the girls. Twigs or rock salt may be inserted into the vagina to maintain a small opening to allow urine and menstrual fluid to pass through and the whole area may be covered with soil and bark at the end of the procedure to promote healing.

As a consequence of the conditions there is no facility for adequately controlling excessive bleeding, e.g. diathermy or appropriate suturing, and significant haemorrhage may occur. Due to uncontrollable bleeding the girls may go in to hypovolemic shock and due to the environment there are usually not the facilities for adequate resuscitation. This may therefore be a pre-terminal event. Generally speaking there is no form of anaesthesia and this is a very painful procedure, which is exaggerated by being forcibly held down and the use of crude instruments.

Intermediate complications

As the environment is not surgically sterile the rate of infection is high and the use of bark and soil significantly increases the risk of developing tetanus and overwhelming sepsis. Due to the nature of the procedure itself the girl may go into urinary retention, or this may be as a consequence of haematoma formation or swelling around the site of the procedure. There is a mortality rate associated with FGM but as the majority of cases are not officially reported there is no figure available for this and one can only rely on anecdotal evidence in a few cases.

Long-term complications

As a result of FGM the stitched area may be completely scarred, leaving no opening for the menstrual blood to be released (haematocolpos). This can result in gross distension of the vagina, which may present as an abdominal mass. This requires surgical correction and opening up of the labia to allow the fluid to escape. Sometimes girls may be killed by parents or family members, believing that the abdominal mass has been caused through pregnancy, suggesting that their daughters have had sexual intercourse before marriage.

Scarring and keloid formation are very common and might relate to the conditions under which the operation was performed and what materials were used (but not necessarily). Keloid formation happens frequently, as the suturing occurs in the midline and often in black women, who are most at risk of keloid formation.

If only a small orifice has been left following FGM, then urine accumulates in the vagina and very gradually drips out. It may take 20–30 minutes for a woman to complete micturition. The stasis of the urine in the narrow, possibly scarred, vagina can lead to recurrent urinary tract infections.

Vulval epidermoid cysts can occur as a direct consequence of FGM and can grow to a significant size, necessitating surgical excision (*see* 9, colour plate section). A longer-term consequence of these cysts is that they may become infected and develop into ulcers.

Vulval abscess is a localised collection of pus that can form on either side of the vulva, as a direct consequence of the operation.

Due to the nature of the conditions of the original procedure, if the external genitalia become infected, this can progress to an ascending infection involving the fallopian tubes and the pelvis. This leads to pyrexia, significant pelvic pain and a foul-smelling discharge. This requires aggressive antibiotic therapy but may result in damage to the fallopian tubes, which might lead to long-term sterility.

A woman may experience pain during the menstrual cycle (dysmenorrhoea), particularly if there is a haematocolpos, as the mass will increase with every cycle and this may also increase the possibility of developing endometriosis through retrograde menstruation.

Sexual dysfunction

It is inevitable that having undergone FGM a woman's genital region will be associated with pain and trauma. This may mean that even if the FGM has resulted in minimal physical damage the sexual response is often decreased or absent. If the clitoris has been removed then orgasm is impossible.

Most women who have had FGM 3 have problems with penetration following marriage. Sometimes the scar tissue is so thick that penetration is impossible and the scarring may lead to either re-cutting (this is traditionally done on the night of her wedding) or forced penetration leading to perineal lacerations. If penetration is impossible then anal intercourse may become the substitute, which can lead to 'fistulae' and fissures, and faecal incontinence.

Many women who had previously had FGM are now seeking reversal of the operation once they wish to become sexually active or when they are pregnant (anticipating a vaginal delivery). The reversal procedure can be done under local or general anaesthesia and involves a vertical incision dividing the previously sutured labia. After dividing the labia, clitoral tissue may be felt or revealed anteriorly, if the original operation had not involved partial or complete removal of the clitoris.

Pelvic examinations

If women present to their general practitioner with pelvic pain, vaginal discharge or request for a cervical smear this may be impossible depending on the degree of FGM that had been performed. These women are unable to have either a bi-manual examination or a trans-vaginal scan, which makes assessment of any gynaecological complaint very difficult.

FGM and early pregnancy problems

As one only needs a pinhole opening for sperm to penetrate into the vagina, and subsequently into the uterus, pregnancy is possible. If any early pregnancy problems occur then they are very difficult to assess for the above reasons. If the woman does go on to have a miscarriage then the foetus may be retained in the vagina with expulsion unable to occur because of the rigid perineum. This can lead to overwhelming infection with serious sequelae of sepsis, shock and death.

Labour

In labour a vaginal examination may not be possible so it is very difficult to assess the progress of labour. The rigid scar tissue may lead to a prolonged and obstructed second stage with subsequent perineal tearing, haemorrhage, fistulae formation, failure to progress, uterine rupture, uterine prolapse, foetal compromise or foetal and/or maternal death.

If women present in labour with FGM 3, this should be reversed early in labour to enable invasive procedures such as vaginal examinations, or foetal blood sampling in case of foetal distress, and to facilitate spontaneous vaginal delivery.

Sometimes FGM is traditionally performed in labour, as it is felt that if a woman has not had FGM and then has a vaginal delivery the baby will be stillborn if it touches the clitoris. If FGM is performed in labour the risks of haemorrhage and death are high.

Post-partum

If reversal has been performed appropriately in labour then there should not be any significant post-partum complications, but if a Caesarean section has occurred then the lochia may collect in the vagina, leading to infection and puerperal sepsis.

Psychological effects

Women who have had FGM often have low self-esteem and feel denied of their sexuality, which is made much worse with the cultural emphasis on reproduction. They often have a genital phobia and may suffer from flashbacks and anxiety, and are at high risk of suicide. Psychological problems are exacerbated if circumcision takes place in an older girl or when the woman is old enough to be fully aware of what is being done to her.

There are significant complications, both physical and psychological, associated with FGM. It is heartening that women are being offered reversal of their FGM at their request so that they are able to use vaginal tampons, have penetrative intercourse, and have normal vaginal deliveries. It is essential that counselling is available pre and post reversal procedure.

The role of the midwife

The Royal College of Midwives (RCM) Position Paper 21[10] outlines the role of the midwife as being to provide the best possible care for each woman, including her physical, emotional, psychosexual, cultural and social needs. This involves the following:

- **Being aware, being informed:** Maternity services should take steps to become aware of local minority ethnic communities which support FGM, and of the special needs of women within those communities. That means talking directly to the communities concerned.
- **Being sensitive, not superior:** It is crucial that midwives do not sound disgusted or patronising when discussing FGM with women from communities which support it. This is an integral part of providing care in a woman-centred, holistic way. Do not make assumptions about the woman's own views. Remember that condescending and racist attitudes, disruption of cultural identity and denial of community values damage women as surely as FGM does.
- **Assessing individual needs:** Midwives should ask, as part of routine antenatal care to the communities concerned, if they have been circumcised. This should be put carefully but directly; a good lead question is 'I understand that female circumcision is usual in your country, have you been cut down here?' If they have, the nature of circumcision and the physical sequelae should be assessed and if necessary the woman should be referred to a specialist, gynaecologist or obstetrician, preferably a female with experience in this area. All women who have been circumcised may appreciate the opportunity to discuss its

implications for their physical and emotional well-being: referral to a specialist support group, or to a psychosexual therapist, may be needed.

- **Informing and explaining:** At all stages of maternity care, women should understand what is happening to them and why. This is particularly important for women who have been circumcised, who may need the services of a skilled interpreter (who should not be a friend or relative). Where a woman has been infibulated, she must be told why de-infibulation is necessary, and why she cannot be re-stitched.
- **Involving partners and families:** It is vital to involve the communities concerned in tackling the problem of FGM, in order to maintain the status and self-esteem of women (particularly women who have been de-infibulated), and to enhance the motivation of both women and men in working to eradicate the practice.
- **Involving and informing other care professionals:** There is a range of other professionals who the midwife may need to involve in maternity care for circumcised women. The consultant obstetrician should be informed of her needs and of any services or referrals undertaken; liaison with the health visitor and GP should ensure seamless postnatal support. If the baby is female, and the family support FGM, social services should be involved and the aim is to support the family to change their attitude, *not* to take the child away from the family. The woman must know who has been informed, and why.
- **Providing continuing support:** Postnatally, the woman should be offered continuing support with any physical and psychological complications arising from FGM and/or deinfibulation.

There have been a number of studies which have sought to establish the quality of maternity services in the UK. Responses are mixed; some women stated that they were happy with the services provided but others gave evidence of shortfalls in the performance of service providers. They cited examples of staff being insensitive to their needs and a lack of information available about healthcare during pregnancy, childbirth and the postnatal period. There is agreement between users and providers that there need to be more interpreters available to explain choices available to women who have little or no English and who do not want family members translating for them. There were, regrettably, examples where women with FGM faced racism and stereotypical attitudes amongst maternity staff. Overall, evidence suggests a lack of consistency in professional practice by maternity services.

Ethical issues and dilemmas

There are some who hold the view that medicalisation of FGM is preferable to women and girls being subjected to the alternative – that is, being mutilated in unclean conditions by untrained traditional attendants using scissors, pieces of glass or razor blades. Whilst at first, one might have some sympathy for this view, it must be clear that most national and international organisations and healthcare bodies agree that health professionals must not carry out FGM, as it runs against basic ethics of healthcare and condones this harmful practice.

Even when families are aware of the illegality of practice of FGM in the UK, they may try to find a traditional circumciser from their own community to perform the procedure on their daughters. It is rare for medically qualified person-nel to be asked to perform FGM, though sadly there are still a few unscrupulous practitioners willing to carry out the procedure for the right price. However, obstetricians and midwives might be asked to re-infibulate a woman following vaginal delivery and it must be explained to them that re-infibulation is not permitted by law in the UK.

Both the RCM and the Royal College of Obstetricians and Gynaecologists (RCOG) make it clear that re-stitching of a previously infibulated woman after vaginal delivery may only be carried out to repair a perineum or vulva which has torn or been cut to facilitate delivery, but not to a degree that makes intercourse difficult or impossible. The law permits surgical operation on the vulva on the grounds of the patient's mental health, but not solely for the purpose of custom or ritual.[10]

The African Well Woman's Clinic

In response to the significant increase in the number of women and girls with FGM attending maternity, gynaecology and family planning clinics, in September 1997 the African Well Woman's Clinic was set up at Guy's and St Thomas' Foundation Trust to support women and girls in the community who have under-gone FGM. All professionals, non-governmental organisations, other organisa-tions and women and girls themselves can refer to the clinic and the working arrangements of the clinic are sufficiently flexible to suit each woman and cater to their individual needs.

The One-stop Clinic is available to women requiring counselling and advice, and they can have their circumcision reversed (with local anaesthetic for pregnant and non-pregnant women), all on the same day. Most importantly, the clinic offers links with the community, facilitates autonomy and empowerment and offers train-ing to GPs, midwives, nurses and other health and social care professionals, as well as local, national and international non-healthcare professionals.

All health and social care professionals have a duty of care and responsibility to protect children who are at risk of FGM. They also have a professional obligation, as part of their continuing development, to read and update themselves on the literature about FGM in relation to cultural/historical background, legal issues, actual and potential short- and long-term complications, FGM and pregnancy and labour and the principles to be followed when FGM is suspected or has been performed.[11]

> Female genital mutilation is a fundamental human rights issue with adverse health and social implications ... [it] violates the rights of girls and women to bodily integrity and results in perpetuating gender inequality.
> UK All Party Parliamentary Group on Population, Development and Reproductive Health

References

1 McCaffrey M, Jankowska A and Gordon H (1995) Management of female genital mutilation: the Northwick Park hospital experience. *Br J Obstet Gynaecol.* **102**: 787–90.

2 Anonymous (1995) Female genital mutilation (Council Report). *JAMA*. **274**: 1714–16.

3 Baker CA, Gilson GJ MD and Curet LB (1993) Female circumcision: obstetric issues. *Am J Obstet Gynecol*. **169**: 1616–18.

4 Lightfoot-Klein H and Shaw E (1991) Special needs of ritually circumcised women patients. *J Obstet Gynecol Neonatal Nursing*. **20**: 102–7.

5 Momoh C, Ladhani S, Lochrie P and Rymer J (2001) Female genital mutilation: analysis of the first twelve months of a southeast London specialist clinic. *British Journal of Obstetrics and Gynaecology*. **108**: 186–91.

6 Lockhat H (2004) *Female Genital Mutilation: treating the tears*. Middlesex University Press, Middlesex.

7 Burnett A and Peel M (2001) Health needs of asylum seekers and refugees. *BMJ*. **322**: 544–7.

8 British Medical Association (BMA) (2002) *Asylum Seekers: meeting their healthcare needs*. BMA, London.

9 Momoh C (2003) Tackling the taboo. *Nursing Times*. **99**, 15: Feature. **15 April**: 40–1.

10 The Royal College of Midwives (RCM) *Position Paper No 21 Female Genital Mutilation (Female Circumcision)*. RCM, London.

11 Momoh C (2005) Female genital mutilation: more common than you think. *Nursing in Practice*: **January–February**: 57–9.

Chapter Four

Female genital mutilation: a clinician's experience

Harry Gordon

Introduction

Various forms of female mutilation are practised worldwide – but mainly in Africa, where at least 28 countries are involved.[1] Traditional circumcisers usually carry out these operations, which leads to individual variation; however, a broad classification has been suggested by the World Health Organization, and is shown in Table 4.1. The most common form of mutilation is FGM 2, which probably accounts for around 80% of all cases.

It is only within the last decade that FGM has assumed clinical importance in Western Europe. This is because civil war and widespread natural disasters in the Horn of Africa have led to immigration by refugees from that area. They practise FGM 3, the most severe form of mutilation, where a barrier is created at the introitus by suturing raw tissues across the mid line after excision of the labia and clitoris. This leaves only a small posterior opening (about 1 cm in diameter or less) (*see* 7, colour plate section).

The main areas where FGM 3 is practised differ from other countries where the other forms of FGM are common in that FGM 3 in the Horn of Africa (especially in Somalia and the Sudan) involves nearly all women (over 90%) and is independent of social class. Where nearly 100% of women have been circumcised, the procedure and its aftermath become accepted as 'part of being a woman'. This

Table 4.1 WHO classification of genital mutilation

Type	Synonym	Extent
FGM 1	Sunna	Removal of clitoris or clitoral hood.
FGM 2	Excision	Removal of clitoris and part of labia.
FGM 3	Infibulation	
Pharaonic circumcision	Removal of clitoris and labia and suture of raw tissues to occlude all but a small area of the introitus	
FGM 4	Various e.g. Gishiri cuts	Pricking, cutting, insertion of corrosives into the vagina (often as a spurious therapeutic measure).

may explain the lack of psychosexual problems encountered in most European clinics dealing with FGM. Surprisingly, in a study of 1836 Ibo women in Nigeria,[2] removal of the clitoris and/or labia (FGM 2) did not attenuate sexual feelings. It did not appear to reduce early arousal during intercourse, or the proportion achieving orgasm.

Clinical presentation

In Europe, doctors see predominantly FGM 3. Why is this when overall FGM 2 (excision) is more common and we have many immigrants from West Africa? The reasons are, first, that no barrier is created at the introitus, and women surviving FGM 2 and 1 are usually asymptomatic – thus even if mutilation is present, it may be overlooked. Second, even in areas with traditionally high levels of FGM only about 45% of women have been circumcised[2] and the long-term morbidity is low. In West Africa, the prevalence of FGM 2 is decreasing with age, social class and the standard of education.[3]

In their study, none of the mothers aged 16–20 had been circumcised.[4] In a 10-year period, only 39 cases of post-circumcision (FGM 2) vulval complications (late complications) were admitted to University College Hospital in Ibadan, Nigeria.[4] This contrasts sharply with the situation in Khartoum, where 7% of the total obstetric and gynaecological operations in Khartoum North Hospital were to treat the direct complications of female circumcision (FGM 3).[5]

In Europe, FGM presents mainly in one of two ways. Either the woman has just married and it has proved impossible to consummate the marriage because of the barrier of scar tissue, or she has become pregnant despite the barrier at the introitus and has an obstruction at the introitus, which will complicate delivery.

In Somalia, if penetrative sex is impossible, de-infibulation (opening up) is carried out by a local midwife or traditional birth attendant immediately after marriage (especially in Northern Somalia, where the residual opening tends to be very small – 0.5 cm or less). If the opening permits, the opening may be widened by forceful penile penetration.[6] These issues have to be addressed in terms of NHS provision. The pregnant woman with an intact circumcision in pregnancy needs special attention and training if staff involved.

Apart from the main presentations, women who have intact FGM 3 may present with other gynaecological and urological complaints. Such cases may have problems because of the difficulty of access for examination. For example, urine will always be contaminated with vaginal organisms and the urethra may not be accessible for catheterisation. Speculum examination may be impossible.[7]

Ethical, religious and legal issues

Whilst Islam is the main religion in areas where FGM is practised, female circumcision is not part of the Islamic faith, and it is not a religious duty. Christian, Jewish and traditional religious groups have also practised circumcision and, conversely, in some Islamic countries such as Pakistan, female genital mutilation is extremely uncommon.

Whilst FGM is now illegal in the UK and most Western countries (Prevention of Circumcision Act 1985 and the recent update 2004), it is important to realise that in the UK re-closure to recreate a barrier at the introitus is also not permitted. In Somalia, re-infibulation is not usually requested. In the Sudan it is commonly carried out after delivery, and Sudanese women may request re-suture and must be told that it is illegal.

Other issues may emerge. One of the commonest is the insistence on only seeing a female doctor. This is not completely true. The requirement is in general to see a female. However, if a male doctor has greater experience in the subject of the consultation then it is a religious duty to see the more experienced doctor, irrespective of gender. Over 10 years of working in clinics for Somali women, we have not found this to be a serious problem.

Within Islam, it is the primary duty of a woman to care for her health and welfare. Sexual intercourse is not permitted during menstruation and other vaginal bleeding. After confinement, intercourse is not permitted for the first 15–40 days after delivery, depending on the health of the mother.

In general, contraception is not permitted. For example, tubal ligation is not acceptable, but there are grey areas in that you can assist a women to have a 'rest' between pregnancies in the interests of her health – i.e. family spacing is acceptable. Termination of pregnancy is not permitted. The fast during Ramadan is a religious duty. The fast can be delayed by sickness, travel and pregnancy. However, the fast must be undertaken at a later date. Most women elect to fast with their family when pregnant.

The fast ends at sundown, and its impact depends on the time of year (Ramadan is not constant in date). If sundown is early, there is little problem, but with increasing hours of daylight, maternal faintness may occur, and there is also indirect evidence of an adverse effect on the foetus.[8] The main problem for medical staff relates to medication, as the timing of oral preparations need to be adjusted, as they cannot be taken during the fast. In the absence of direct instruction, women may use inappropriate time intervals or, worse still, they may omit the medication.

Recreational drugs and alcohol are not permitted. Overall, the important message is that when dealing with a defined religious group in the community, it is important for staff to have a basic knowledge of any situations that can affect treatment. It is also important to avoid advice which may be offensive. In our experience with Muslim women it is in the area of family planning that medical and nursing staff are most likely to inadvertently cause offence.

Advice in planning services for women with FGM 3

Within the National Health Service in the UK there are problems that have to be addressed. Many of these are common to all immigrant populations who are fleeing from areas of serious civil unrest. Some problems are specific to women who have suffered genital mutilation, especially FGM 3.

General problems

The refugees from war areas are normally biased in social class, with a deficiency in lower social classes. This relates to the need to provide bribes, and to have enough cash reserves to pay their way out of the country. There is also a bias towards the young and fit. The language barrier is an obvious problem, and as the host language is learned, medical terminology is not usually developed. This leads to a potentially dangerous situation. The women may attend a doctor and apparently speak good social English. However, medical terminology may be misunderstood and a grossly misleading history may be obtained.

It is also important to find how each community obtains its information on health matters. For the Somali community, word of mouth is extremely important – more important than any other form of communication. Health authorities may waste money on leaflets and videos, which have little impact. Somalia in the past had a Northern area, which was an English colony, and the South was an Italian colony, and most educated Somalis will be familiar with one or other language – this also defines area of choice for immigrants.

Specific medical issues

Our experience in West London has shown a relatively high incidence of tuberculosis, including extra pulmonary lesions. Hepatitis B carriers also occur relatively frequently (7%). A few women may carry the scars of war (bullet wounds and burns). HIV positive cases are in our experience rare in Somali women. We have only had one case in over 10 years.

Issues relating to genital mutilation

Women who present in pregnancy or with medical problems will not mention circumcision unless asked. Talk of 'mutilation' will be offensive, and simple terms such as 'are you open or closed', or 'have you been circumcised' are understood, and are acceptable. Once it is established that FGM has taken place, examination is essential to determine the extent of damage. Do not rely on what the woman says, as they may be unaware of the extent of damage. It is not uncommon for the woman to say, 'I only have Sunna' (FGM 1) when on examination extensive FGM 3 is identified. Conversely, we see women who admit to being circumcised and on examination are normal.

Apart from the physical barrier at the introitus, about 5% of women will have associated epidermal cysts. These may reach a considerable size, and usually arise in the paraclitoral area. However, on average they are quite small ($\pm$1 cm) but they may cause symptoms if they become infected, or if there is haemorrhage into the cyst. We have also seen dyspareunia and pain on orgasm related to small cysts, which had not been removed at the time of de-infibulation.

Suggested guidelines for NHS services

Where there is a significant population of women likely to have been circumcised (e.g. London, Liverpool, Cardiff, Sheffield, Manchester and Birmingham), serious consideration should be given to establishing a specific clinic for these mainly Somali women. The clinic should involve a consultant with an interest in the subject and two senior midwives. A reliable translator is extremely important. She (a female is essential in this role) should be reliable and of an age and social class acceptable to the community. This appointment is important for the success of the clinic and provides an invaluable link into the community. This involvement of a named consultant ensures that all complications can be dealt with without delay, and without unnecessary internal referrals. Two midwives are needed to ensure continued expertise at times of holidays and illness.

The ethnic origin of the midwives is not relevant – though a Somali or Arabic speaker is convenient it is not essential. The clinic as set up can deal with obstetric and gynaecological problems, as well as women seeking primary de-infibulation. The only true cost is the translator and in any case the provision of adequate interpretation is an NHS requirement. These women will attend the hospital in any case, and the clinic will ensure that they are dealt with efficiently and their problems are understood. It also ensures efficient use of the interpreter's time. Use of children and male relatives, as interpreters, should be avoided.

Each clinic should develop its own protocols, depending on experience and the local situation. The protocols we use at the Central Middlesex Hospital[9] may help hospitals that are intent on providing a clinic service.

Essentially there are four groups of women who need provision.

1 **Women who are not pregnant and wish reversal of circumcision:** Examination in the clinic should be brief, usually just looking at the area with no attempt at internal examination, which is pointless in terms of adequate clinical assessment, may be painful and may in some cases precipitate distressing 'flashback' memories of the original procedure. Gentle palpation in the clitoral area may provide evidence of normal clitoral tissue under the scar tissue. We have found 70% of cases have an intact and normal clitoris under the scar[10] (*see* 8, colour plate section).

   It is important to provide facilities for operation without delay, remembering that most of these women are recently married and are unable to consummate the union. Delay is cruel and causes distress and marital disharmony. You should be able to guarantee operation within a month at the very most. All the operations can be carried out as day care procedures.

   We in West London offer a choice of anaesthesia, general, local or spinal. Our patients seem averse to local anaesthesia, and most requests are for a general anaesthetic. This is unlike the experience at St Thomas' Hospital in South London, where most cases are de-infibulation under local anaesthesia, most at the time of first clinic attendance. Clearly, local communities vary in their attitude to anaesthesia (Momoh 2000, personal communication). Certainly a one stop clinic has much to commend it.

2 **Women who are pregnant with an intact circumcision:** Our policy is designed to ensure that as few women as possible present in labour with the circumcision intact. It is stressful for the midwife and dangerous for the woman if the midwife and/or junior doctor are unfamiliar with the technique for de-infibulation. Whilst you can institute a regular training programme, the turnover of midwives and junior doctors means that there is still a significant risk of the labouring women encountering staff who do not understand what to do. Delay may result in serious perineal damage.

   In these circumstances, we have seen the women subjected to a wide episiotomy, in an attempt to deliver the foetal head behind the scar. We have also seen women who have had a bilateral episiotomy, which is very damaging to perineal function and should never be employed.

All these problems can be avoided if the circumcision is opened up in the antenatal period. We advise reversal under local or spinal anaesthesia between 18 and 24 weeks of pregnancy. This avoids the time when miscarriage is common, as if it were to occur following a reversal procedure, the woman would assume that the operation had caused the miscarriage. 18–24 weeks also tends to be a time of 'obstetric tranquillity'.

When we introduced this policy at Northwick Park Hospital, the community accepted it, and only 14% of reversals were carried out in labour.[10] When the clinic transferred to serve a more deprived population at the Central Middlesex Hospital, we found a greater reluctance to accept antenatal reversal, and 60% opted to await the onset of labour. This was at least in part due to the mistaken assumption that they would inevitably need an episiotomy 'so why not combine both reversal and episiotomy – in one procedure'.

In fact, after antenatal reversal the woman has a good chance of delivering with an intact perineum. If the infibulation is left intact, remember that most urine samples are contaminated with vaginal secretions, and it is difficult to determine the significance of proteinurea. It is important that the state of the perineum is described in the antenatal notes and that clear written instructions on de-infibulation are included.

If a woman slips through the net, and presents for the first time in labour with an intact circumcision, this can be very frightening for an inexperienced midwife. In fact, resolution of the situation is simple. The scar should be infiltrated with local anaesthetic, and incised in the mid line until the urethra is exposed. This allows maximum room for delivery and avoids the potentially vascular clitoral area. Significant bleeding is rarely encountered, and suture can be left until after delivery. If there are any troublesome bleeding points, they can be oversewn. Where a circumcised woman requires elective or emergency Caesarean section, try to obtain permission to carry out de-infibulation under the same anaesthetic.

3 **Women who are pregnant for the second or subsequent time:** Somali women are not usually re-sutured, and are therefore likely to be open. In the Sudan, re-infibulation is almost universal. Whatever the ethnic group, the perineum should be examined to exclude abnormal scarring, or formation of adhesions.

4 Women who have a primary gynaecological complaint unrelated to the genital mutilation may require de-infibulation to facilitate examination.[6]

Surgical technique

Surgery is simple, and can be carried out on a day care basis. Where elective surgery is carried out, the scar should be incised strictly in the mid line. The clitoris and clitoral hood are present in most cases, buried under the scar tissue. The only point to remember is that the distance from the urethra to the base of the clitoris varies from 1 cm to 5 cm, so an adequate extension of the incision beyond the urethra is needed before you can assume that the clitoris has been removed.

Other issues

Family planning

This is an important issue, and attendance at a routine family planning clinic is rarely successful. There are often language difficulties, and the advice given may conflict with the woman's religious duties.[11] There are several ways of overcoming this problem. A family planning ward round of the postnatal ward with the interpreter will help a number of women. However, this is likely to occur no more frequently than weekly, and many women may be missed.

A family planning nurse could attend the clinic where postnatal examinations are carried out and advice can be given. However, default from this clinic is common. The best option is to provide added training for those providing family planning advice and to ensure that at least one main clinic provides an interpreter.

For this population, high parity is prized, and is regarded as more important than social or financial considerations. Family planning must therefore concentrate most on family spacing. In our West London Clinic, the mean parity is five and parity up to 10 not uncommon.

General issues related to pregnancy

Although some African papers have suggested a high perinatal mortality related to genital mutilation,[12,13] it is quite clear that in a European context there is no association between FGM and perinatal death.[14]

Somali women do not like Caesarean sections or induction of labour, and when advised, careful explanation needs to be given or the woman, if she disagrees with your advice, may default from antenatal care and only reappear in labour. High parity in this population does not seem to carry the same dangers as those suggested in a European population – almost certainly because high parity is achieved at a surprisingly young age in Somali women, and delivery tends to be uncomplicated. This may well affect decisions about delivery in a low-risk birthing unit.

Conclusion

Knowledge of the management of FGM and provision of services that provide amongst other things adequate interpretation can reduce the problems of this population to the minimum, and deliver perinatal mortality at least close to European standards.

References

1 Dorkenoo E (1995) *Cutting the Rose. Female genital mutilation: the practice and its prevention.* Minority Rights Publications, London.
2 Onkonofua FB, Larsen U, Oronsaye F *et al.* (2002) The association between female genital cutting and corelatus of sexual and gynaecological morbidity in Edo State Nigeria. *British Journal of Obstetrics and Gynaecology.* **109**: 1089–96.
3 Igwegbe AO and Egbuonu I (2000) The prevalence and practice of female genital mutilation in Nnewi, Nigeria: The impact of female education. *Journal of Obstetrics and Gynaecology.* **20**: 520–22.

4 Adekunle AO, Fakokkunde A, Odukogbe A *et al.* (1999) Female genital mutilation post circumcision vulval complications in Nigerians. *Journal of Obstetrics and Gynaecology.* **19**: 632–5.

5 Mawad NM and Hassanein OM (1994) Female circumcision, three years' experience of common complications in patients treated in Khartoum teaching hospitals. *Journal of Obstetrics and Gynaecology.* **14**: 40–43.

6 McCaffrey M, Jankowska A and Gordon H (1995) Management of female genital mutilation: the Northwick Park Hospital experience. *British Journal of Obstetrics and Gynaecology.* **102**: 787–90.

7 Baker CA, Gilson GJ, Vill HD *et al.* (1993) Female circumcision: obstetric issues. *American Journal of Obstetrics and Gynaecology.* **169**: 1616–18.

8 Mirghani SD, Weerasinghe SD, Smith JR *et al.* (2004) The effect of intermittent maternal fasting on human foetal breathing movements. *Journal of Obstetrics and Gynaecology.* **24**: 635–7.

9 Gordon H *et al.* (2005) Experience of the last 5 years of a West London clinic for women with FGM. *Journal of Obstetrics and Gynaecology* [in press].

10 Gordon H (1998) Female genital mutilation. *The Diplomate.* **5**: 86–90.

11 Comerasamy H, Read B, Francis C *et al.* (2003) The acceptability and use of contraception: a prospective study of Somalian women's attitude. *Journal of Obstetrics and Gynaecology.* **23**: 412–15.

12 De Silva S (1989) Obstetric sequel of female circumcision. *European Journal of Obstetrics, Gynaecology and Reproductive Biology.* **32**: 233–40.

13 Berardi JC, Teillet TF, Laloux V *et al.* (1985) Obstetric consequences of female circumcision. *Journal of Gynaecology, Obstetrics and Reproductive Biology.* **14**: 743–46.

14 Essen B, Bödker B, Sjöberg N-O *et al.* (2002) Is there an association between female circumcision and perinatal death. *Bulletin of the World Health Organization.* **80**: 629–32.

Chapter Five

Care of circumcised young women and girls

Nahid Toubia

Background

The circumcision of a child may be discovered accidentally, as a result of a medical check-up or treatment for a common childhood illness. External to the clinical environment, a teacher, immigration caseworker or social worker, for example, may come into contact with a child or adolescent who displays physical and/or psychological symptoms of having undergone female circumcision. The police service or other authorities might encounter such cases in the course of investigations into breaches of national laws relating to prohibition of the practice inside their borders.

Finding oneself observing the circumcised genitalia of a child or adolescent for the first time may well stir up strong feelings of shock, disbelief, revulsion or sadness, for example, emotions even more powerful because of the age and innocence of the victim. Whilst such responses may be understandable, it must be remembered that those who submit their daughters to female circumcision believe it to be a culturally normalised procedure that is in the best interests of the child, and not cruel abuse, as perceived in the West.

It is most likely that a child's family will have gone to great lengths and made significant financial sacrifice to provide what they see as their daughter's rite of passage into womanhood and are likely to be loving, rather than violent, parents. It is important that the family is treated with respect and their right to privacy ensured. Confrontational exchanges would have no tangible benefits for the child, family or service providers involved.

The girl was probably circumcised before emigrating with her family from her homeland. However, given the increasing flow of immigrants and refugees from countries where female circumcision (FC) is prevalent, some girls may have been circumcised just before arrival in the host country, having heard that the practice is illegal here. As circumcision may have been performed, or its complications become apparent, very recently, there may be difficulty in determining where the procedure took place.

If the procedure has been performed in the host country, it is illegal under criminal statute and therefore may be reportable under child abuse or child protection legislation. This is the case in all Western countries regardless of whether there is a specific FC/FGM law; the perpetrator(s) might also be prosecuted for assault/bodily harm. If FGM has been performed prior to arrival in host country, it is outside the jurisdiction of the receiving country and is probably not reportable since no further harm to the child is likely. If, however, there are younger female siblings in the family, service providers may well infer that younger children are at risk and that reporting is warranted.

If a delivered mother has a girl child, some healthcare providers will be faced with a request from her or her family to circumcise the daughter. Confusion has arisen in the US when nurses refuse to circumcise the baby girl but agree to or even offer a circumcision for a baby boy. Should such a situation arise, healthcare workers should use this as an opportunity to educate the family and help protect the child; a hostile reaction or attempt to dismiss the request is unhelpful.

The best course of action is to first acknowledge that you know that female circumcision is a tradition performed in their culture but go on to say that there have been many studies and information from African countries to show that this practice is harmful to girls and women. In view of this, the practice has been made illegal and anyone performing female circumcision in the UK, US or any other Western nation would be breaking the law and could be jailed or deported (if a foreign national).

When holding a conversation with the parents, make it clear that you under-stand where the family is coming from and make clear that you will not condemn or judge them for asking you. Discuss with them the adjustments that they have all had to make to a society where the culture is very different. Emphasise the harmful effects of FC/FGM on the girl's physical, mental and sexual health now, within marriage, and beyond to childbearing.

If parents mention sending the child to their country of origin to be circumcised, remind them that they are putting their daughter through tremendous and unnecessary physical risk. Bring to their attention that they are in a new country and their daughter could grow up feeling different from her uncircumcised friends. In addition, reinforce the message that they can still be prosecuted under the law if they return to the host country having had their child circumcised elsewhere.

The protection of the child must remain paramount. Stress the point that FC/FGM is not a requirement of any religion, though it might be interpreted as being so by some individuals or local religious leaders; explain that there are other ways of maintaining a cultural heritage. If the provider is unable to counsel the parents themselves they should refer them to a counsellor trained in this matter.

However sensitive you may be in your interaction with families, they may well become bewildered and confused by what you are telling them. Provide them with written literature on the health, religious and legal aspects of FC/FGM if you have them and any information on local community organisations working against the practice. This will reinforce the verbal message and should be available where possible in their native language.

There is no substantive proof that adolescent girls, living in a new country and who have been circumcised, experience particular problems associated with FC/FGM. However, there is enough anecdotal evidence to suggest that their concerns about circumcision are entwined with other issues faced by most teenage girls all over the world regarding sexual image, attractiveness, identity, belonging and conforming with their peers.

These girls may or may not have known that they had been circumcised while in their home country. Surrounded by a family unit who would never consider open discussion of such matters, it might not have crossed their minds. On arrival in the host country things might be very different. They have reached the age where they have become inquisitive about their bodies. They may have heard about FC/FGM in the liberal Western media, and started to wonder if they have had the ritual performed on them. Vague memories of a childhood experience could begin to take on a new meaning.

A healthcare practitioner may become aware that a girl has been circumcised quite by chance, during sexual health education by a school nurse or practice nurse giving contraceptive counselling for instance. She may voluntarily disclose that she has been circumcised to a medical practitioner. Whatever the circumstances, the professional must listen and not assume that the young woman has revealed this information because she is having related problems.

She may have accepted FC/FGM as a part of her cultural heritage and not be troubled by it; a peer support group might be a mechanism for providing her to share experiences with other girls who have been circumcised. Professionals must avoid making them feel in any way 'different' from their peers, as to do so would jeopardise the relationship and might trigger worries in the teenager when engaging with family and friends. Whatever the reason for her disclosure, she should be afforded the same access to professional advice and support afforded to all other teenagers.

Alternatively, an adolescent girl may confide in you that she wishes to embark on a sexual relationship or seeks advice about physical problems, which may or may not be linked to FC/FGM and need attention. Those young women who have been infibulated may request de-infibulation. For healthcare professionals, this raises issues of adolescents' privacy and safety and the ethical-legal questions that arise regarding provision of such services to a minor without parental consent. Very careful, thorough consideration must be given to the professional repercussions, and these must be balanced with the health and well-being of the young person and her subsequent relationship with her family.

Arguably the greatest dilemma for these adolescents is coping with the differing values and beliefs of two very different cultures. They naturally feel a strong bond with their roots and the traditional values that discourage sex outside marriage. But they are also drawn to the culture that espouses gender equality, sexual freedom and free will. Tensions may arise within the family when the two cultural perspectives collide. Those trained to facilitate dialogue within families from minority backgrounds must share information with other professionals and lay workers in voluntary organisations to enable development of greater understanding of the practice of FC/FGM and the needs of young people who are or are at risk of becoming victims.

Successful communication

There is probably no better example of a need for cultural awareness than when interacting with women with FC/FGM, and effective communication is crucial. Cultural competence in healthcare has been defined as:

> The ability of individuals and systems to respond respectfully and effectively to people of all cultures, in a manner that affirms the worth and preserves the dignity of individuals, families and communities.[1]

Physicians, nurses and midwives are ideally placed to inform and educate clients about the practice of FC/FGM and empower women to explore their perceptions of themselves, their bodies, reproductive health needs and sense of what they require from healthcare providers. Women must be given choices, as to the extent of obstetric and gynaecology services they require. Some will want standard service provision whilst others may request additional attention to needs associated with FC/FGM.

When holding a two-way dialogue with clients, and in building positive rapport, service providers must be conscious of their own background, values and beliefs systems. They must ensure that they do not allow such factors to influence or impinge on their attitudes towards this client group. The root of successful communication with women and families affected by FC/FGM is for discussion to be probing without being judgemental and for there to be exchange of information on an equitable basis.

Standard documentation, i.e. history-taking forms, do not always take account of the particularly sensitive nature of consultations between women with FC/FGM and healthcare professionals. One must remember that others may have access to paperwork and, as women are unlikely to want details of their FC/FGM to enter the public domain, it is advisable for there not to be FC/FGM-related questions included.

However, it might be felt appropriate to casually ask whether they have had any previous surgery in a 'private' area which the doctor or nurse should know about. It is unlikely that women will be familiar with terminology about FC/FGM and answers to questions like, for instance, the type or extent of circumcision will have to wait until they are examined. That said, care must be taken to avoid terms like 'mutilation' when talking to clients, as they may take offence; the majority of women would be comfortable with 'circumcision'.

Health professionals working in non-specialised areas of clinical practice are unlikely to be exposed to women with FC/FGM on a regular basis. Whilst they may be surprised, during what they thought would be a routine gynaecological examination, it is imperative that they do not display non-verbal signs of disapproval or abhorrence and do not adopt pitying or patronising attitudes.

As aforementioned, those with little or no experience of dealing with women with FC/FGM, and who might not have received any education or training on the practice, could be tempted to share the experience with colleagues. The damage caused by calling in others to view this discovery cannot be overstated and is totally inappropriate. One woman graphically described,

> The feeling of vulnerability and shame I felt lying on my back naked with my legs open and being reduced to a curious spectacle on public display is something I will never forget. It is worse than what I remember of the circumcision.

Never assume that because a woman comes from an African or Middle-Eastern country that she has been circumcised. Neither should you discount the possibility because they are of a religion not usually associated with the practice. Within each culture, religion, region there will be social variations, and labelling should be avoided. Clients should be made to feel welcome; in specialist clinics, acknowledgement of cultures, language and mode of dress goes a long way to making clients feel at ease and is more likely to facilitate open discussion and determine the success of subsequent conversation.

In Western cultures it has become commonplace for women to actively participate in decision making regarding their healthcare and treatment. However, in many African cultures, it is usual for the family to be involved, and the service provider should assess the situation on an individual basis and be respectful and supportive of her choice.

The same applies in respect of clients' perception of what you can provide for them and the issue of traditional medicine. There is research suggesting that some traditional medicine is harmful, but there is also evidence that some remedies are beneficial or pose no danger to the recipient. Commonsense should prevail in such cases; endorsement to those therapies that provide physical and/or psychological comfort, and education to discourage those that are potentially harmful should be the order of the day.

Information should be clear, appropriate and timely. It is important that a client grasps vital information necessary for her to make a decision about treatment and she should be encouraged to ask questions and time should be given for her to interpret information. Immigrant and refugee women identify language as one of the major barriers to accessing healthcare services. Interpreters should be available, where necessary, and use of pictures and diagrams, and literature written in their native language will contribute to effective interaction.

One of the most commonly perceived barriers to communication is that women from non-Western cultures prefer to be seen by a clinician of their own gender. Whilst this may be true in some cases, in others, they may voice more confidence in the wisdom of male physicians. In the case of nurses, midwives and interpreters, it is true that there is a preference for females, as they see them as allies and confidantes. In practice, most circumcised women are drawn to specialist clinics recommended by other women that have the reputation for sensitivity and socio-cultural awareness and empathy, and who are non-discriminatory.

Questions asked by healthcare providers

Practitioners often ask whether or not it is appropriate to talk further with a woman about her circumcision and the answer is, only if it is necessary. This response logically moves on to the question of when it is necessary. If the reason for a woman's attendance at a hospital or clinic is related to FC/FGM – for example, if she presents with complications – then it would obviously be necessary to give an explanation of the cause(s) and what treatment would be required.

If the woman has been infibulated and pregnant, then de-infibulation and the practice of re-infibulation will have to be discussed. If the reason for her attendance is not affected by her circumcision then the matter need not be discussed further, unless the woman herself indicates that she wishes to do so.

There have been occasions when practitioners have felt that circumcised women might benefit from a greater understanding of their genitalia, but this should not be the norm during the first visit and should be used judiciously to avoid women being traumatised by the experience.

It is a fine line between overemphasising the 'difference' with one woman's body to another, and missing an opportunity to talk openly about matters that the woman has indicated she would like to raise. The rule of thumb should be to let the woman know that you are willing and able to discuss any issues with her, but only when she is ready and comfortable doing so.

This chapter has been adapted, with kind permission of the author, from *Caring for Women with Circumcision: A Technical Manual for Health Care Providers* by Nahid Toubia, MD, published by Rainbo 1999.

References

1   Refugee Health Program (1996) *Six Steps Towards Cultural Competence: How to meet the health care needs of immigrants and refugees.* RHP, Minnesota.

Chapter Six

Healthcare provision for pregnant asylum seekers and refugees

Jacqueline Dunkley-Bent

Introduction

Midwives are in a privileged and unique position when providing healthcare to childbearing women. Pregnancy and childbirth can be described as one of the most significant profound experiences in a woman's life cycle, but unfortunately for some it is shadowed by negativity and memories of trauma. Maternity care provision can present many hidden challenges that require flexible, sensitive and discerning qualities when supporting women throughout the childbirth continuum. Providing healthcare in a multicultural society with a migrant population and increasing numbers of asylum seekers and refugees has impacted on the nature of healthcare provision and challenged current practices.

This chapter will highlight some of the issues faced by women who are seeking asylum and refugees who have experienced female genital mutilation (FGM). These women are socially and economically disadvantaged, with health profiles that may be compromised by poor nutrition, torturous journeys from countries of origin and the turmoil of civil war or societal unrest. They require healthcare that is tailored to meet their specific needs. Midwives are at the forefront of planning and delivering care to these women who are at greater risk of severe morbidity.[1]

Unfortunately, inequality in health and healthcare provision continues to exist in the United Kingdom, where disadvantaged and marginalised groups continue to experience poorer health and reduced life expectancy than their counterparts in higher social groups who are economically advantaged. Inequality in health and healthcare provision is explored briefly within this context and the potential for enhancing health through health promotion. The reader is expected to have read the preceding chapters to contextualise the nature of FGM and its origins.

Human rights

All human beings, regardless of age, gender, colour or ethnicity, have the right to physical and mental integrity. This is a basic human right that is guaranteed by international law through the Universal Declaration of Human Rights. In practice this means that women and girls have a right of control over their own bodies. Unfortunately, a woman's freedom to assert this control is often restricted by the threat of social exclusion and the threat of violence exerted by the community and individuals.

Female genital mutilation is an extreme manifestation of violence used to curtail female expression. It also serves to control women, particularly the control of sexuality, which is central to maintaining the subordination of women. The World Health Organization states that two million girls each year are put through the terrifying and painful experience of FGM. Worldwide it is estimated that over 100 million women have been subject to this procedure.[2]

Free healthcare for asylum seekers and refugees?

An *asylum seeker* is a person who has submitted an application for protection under the Geneva Convention and is waiting for the claim to be decided by the Home Office. A *refugee* is a person who has fled their country of origin or is unable to return because he/she fears persecution due to race, religion, nationality, political opinion or membership of a social group. The term 'refugee' is used to describe displaced people all over the world. In the legal context in the UK, a person is a refugee when the Home Office has accepted their asylum claim.

Refugee status means that a person has been accepted under the Geneva Convention and granted indefinite leave to remain, which means permanent residence in the UK.

Britain is a signatory to the 1951 Geneva Convention that is committed to offering asylum to people fleeing persecution. Before the implementation of the Immigration and Asylum Act 1999, the Benefits Agency and local authorities provided support to asylum seekers. From April 2000 the National Asylum Support Service (NASS) took over this service.

NASS are responsible for providing support for all destitute asylum seekers until the Home Office determine their asylum application. Pregnant women receive a maternity grant from NASS worth £300. The application for this grant must be made between 36 weeks gestation and up to two weeks after birth. In addition each adult receives £14 per week and vouchers that can be exchanged for food items. An additional payment of £3 a week has also been introduced to enable expectant mothers to supplement their diet. When NASS receive the new baby's birth certificate the support rate is recalculated to include an additional £38.50 for the new child and also a further £5 with which the mother may purchase baby milk.[3] All asylum seekers and refugees are entitled to full NHS care including dental treatment and registration with a GP.

Most asylum seekers are young men, but worldwide the majority of refugees are women. An application for asylum is usually made at the port of entry, where asylum seekers remain for 10 days in an induction centre. During this time they should apply for NASS support and undergo a health screen check. After 10 days they are dispersed to accommodation centres where they remain for six months, during which time their application is considered.

If the application is turned down, asylum seekers have one right of appeal; if this is rejected, they are transferred to a removal centre in preparation for return to their native country. If the application is successful they are provided with accommodation and integrated into the community. Section 55 of the Asylum Act (2002) allows the denial of benefits to asylum seekers who fail to register their application within three days of arrival.

Approximately 10 000 asylum seekers each year are likely to be made destitute by Section 55 in London.[4] A proportion of these will be pregnant women who may feel unable to speak out on arrival in the UK and complete the application for asylum because they are fearful of the process. Others may have been promised accommodation and support outside of the NASS system by distant family and friends, but very quickly find themselves without any social support and denial of benefits.

Dispersal

Asylum seekers are being dispersed throughout the UK to accommodation centres where health professionals have little experience of working with people from these groups. An appreciation of the trauma experienced in their native countries may be lacking and their expression of pain poorly understood (*see* Box 6.1).

Box 6.1   Problems faced by asylum seekers

Psychological, social and physical problems

Depression, stress, anxiety, fear of people in authority, oppression, persecution, rape, carrying a pregnancy as result of rape, rape during pregnancy, homesickness, separation from family, stress-related physical ill health, deprivation of human rights, political repression, loss of status, harassment, racial harassment, coping with new culture, limited or no access to community network, uncertainty around claiming asylum in the UK, anxiety about the outcome of asylum, fear of deportation, detention, poverty, experiencing guilt and anxiety of those left behind, feelings of insecurity, powerlessness and inability to settle, symptoms of psychological distress, extreme sadness, anxiety, depression, panic attacks, poor concentration.[5]

NB Many people's health deteriorates after arrival; social isolation and poverty have a negative effect on physical and psychological health.

Communicable disease

Tuberculosis
Hepatitis A, B, C
HIV/AIDS
Parasite infections

Effects of war and torture

Partial loss of vision, rape, sexual assault, witnessing death and torture of others, malnutrition, imprisonment, injuries arising from beatings and torture (including dental torture), held under siege, human siege, forcible destruction of home/property.[6] Landmine injuries, amputated limbs, lameness.

Handheld records are vitally important when asylum seekers are dispersed and can facilitate communication to this mobile population. All asylum seekers are issued with health records at the induction centres. Midwives are encouraged to review the health records and complete the appropriate sections detailing pregnancy information and questions on FGM. This section does not detail how to ask the question but simply states 'FGM Yes/No'. Unsurprisingly this section is frequently blank, as disclosing this intimate level of information on arrival in the country can be very difficult. Also, the language used to describe FGM may be alien and or offensive to many women; equally, survivors of further trauma, e.g. torture or rape, may not volunteer this information due to feelings of guilt, shame or mistrust of the authorities.

Health needs

The majority of asylum seeker entrants to the United Kingdom in 2003 were from countries including Iraq, Zimbabwe, Afghanistan and Somalia.[7] FGM is practised in 28 African countries, in South-East Asia and the Middle East. The highest prevalence rates are found in Djibouti, Guinea, Somalia, Eritrea, Mali, Sierra Leone and Sudan. Sudan is cited as having the highest practice in the world.

It is difficult to establish the number of asylum seekers who have undergone FGM, as this information may not be disclosed at the induction centres or may not be identified until labour starts. It is extremely difficult for women to disclose that they have undergone FGM, or even consider discussing it with complete strangers, when there are many other issues and personal needs that cause them greater concern at that time.

Assessing health needs enables the identification of target areas for health promotion work. The health professional's perception of health need may differ from that of the woman. The woman's health needs are varied and are perceived as needs based on subjective criteria. It is suggested that the purpose of need must be justifiable for it to be perceived as a need.[8] The health needs of asylum seekers are multiple, complex and varied. The most efficient way of determining need is a joint discussion and decision between the woman and the health professional.

Maslow's hierarchy of need[9] is a frequently cited model, which shows that all human needs are health needs. The hierarchy suggests that social and economic conditions must first be satisfied before an individual can personally grow to self-actualisation. Basic physiological needs including hunger, thirst and related needs represent the first level of the hierarchy and are usually required to be satisfied before an individual can seek to address higher needs, including:

- safety needs: to feel secure and out of danger
- belongingness and love needs: to affiliate with others, be accepted and belong
- self-esteem needs: to achieve, be competent, gain approval and recognition
- intellectual, aesthetic needs
- self-actualisation needs: to find fulfilment and realise one's own potential.

Asylum seekers frequently strive for safety first, as many physiological needs have been compromised during many months, sometimes years, of oppressive regimes and or torture. Their tolerance during difficult, physically challenging situations is heightened to enable them to reach a place of safety. Women who have experienced severe trauma (*see* Box 6.1) and are pregnant as a result of rape very often continue to feel unsafe and insecure once arriving in the UK, and tend to have low self-esteem.

Making decisions about pregnancy and labour choices can therefore be extremely challenging at this time. They require support that is sensitive, flexible and empathetic. Women may begin to feel safe and have a sense of belonging if their asylum applications have been accepted and they have a place they can call home. Until this time health professionals should be mindful of their vulnerabilities.

On first contact with pregnant asylum seekers midwives should:

- provide timely antenatal care
- assess mental health, as well as physical health (*see* Box 6.1)
- review the patient's health records and record information where appropriate
- encourage registration with a dentist and GP
- book a female interpreter, if necessary (do not use a relative)
- explain the NHS system and further appointments
- explain entitlement to benefits
- link with refugee community organisation
- register with the local Sure Start programme if geographically viable
- if FGM is disclosed, link with FGM specialist or midwife/obstetrician with experience in this area
- use terminology that is culturally appropriate when screening for FGM e.g. Are you closed? Are you open? (Chapter 5 provides further information.)

Seeking asylum status to avoid FGM

A growing number of countries in recent years have granted asylum to women on the grounds that certain acts of violence against women may be considered sufficiently serious to constitute a form of harm amounting to persecution within the meaning of the Refugee Convention (as amended by the 1967 protocol). Gender can influence or even determine both the type of harm inflicted and the reasons for it. Women have been granted asylum because of the risk that they would be subject to female genital mutilation, domestic violence and other serious gender-related harm.

Women sometimes have difficulty presenting their asylum claims because they may be ashamed or afraid to report the violations they have suffered. Unfortunately, immigration officials may not understand the difficulties women have when being asked to recount their experiences of violence, harassment or discrimination. FGM is now regarded as persecution. A woman can be considered a refugee if she or her daughter/s fear being forced to undergo FGM against their will or the mother fears persecution for refusing to let her daughters undergo the procedure.[10]

In 1993 a Somali woman was granted refugee status in Canada after fleeing her country with her 10-year-old daughter, who was at risk of FGM if they returned to their country of origin. In 1996 a woman escaping from Togo because of the threat of FGM was granted asylum status by the United States authorities. In 1997 two families were granted asylum in Sweden on the grounds that the female members of the family would undergo FGM if they returned to Togo, their country of origin.

They were granted residence permits on humanitarian grounds, as the authorities did not recognise them as refugees under the United Nations Refugee Convention. It is important that there is clarity with regards to the recognition of FGM as a form of persecution within the meaning of the Refugee Convention. Disparity and different interpretations of meaning serve only to continue the basic human rights struggle these women face daily.

Protecting children

FGM has been illegal in the UK since the Prohibition of Female Circumcision Act 1985. It was possible for people to undermine the Act by having the procedure performed outside the country. *Working Together to Safeguard Children*[11] highlights that a local authority may exercise its powers under Section 47 of the Children Act 1989 if it has reason to believe that a girl is likely to be, or has been, the subject of FGM. The New 2003 FGM Act strengthens the 1985 Act prohibiting the removal of children from this country to have FGM performed. The FGM Act (2003) that came into force in March 2004 states that it is illegal to take girls abroad for FGM.[12]

All health professionals should be aware of this change in the law and work together to ensure that children are supported and kept safe within family networks. Where a family has been identified as 'at risk' it is important to inform other key services. If the midwife is the first person to identify a family, as being at risk, she should inform the health visitor, the woman's GP and social services.

The midwife, other health professionals and advocacy workers have a responsibility to ensure that the woman and her family understand the new Act, which, if not enforced, can lead to a prison sentence. Midwives must be mindful that despite the severe consequences of FGM, parents and others who wish to do this to their daughters genuinely believe it is in the girls' best interest to conform to the custom. It is not intended as an act of abuse.

Midwives may consider:

- Talking to the family about the health risks outside of the home environment.
- Clear documentation of any discussion and action plans.
- Documentation detailing involvement of other services including action plans.
- If a family disregard advice and information and choose to disengage with health services it will be necessary to ask the police to get a Prohibited Steps Order making it clear to the family that they will be breaking the law if they arrange to have their daughter/s undergo the procedure.
- Continued follow-up with the family until the health visitor is fully engaged.

Health promotion

The provision of health promotion is more meaningful if it is delivered within the context of the individual's everyday life, as the social and economic context of people's lives is closely bound with their health experience.[8] Embracing a victim-blaming ideology with women who have experienced FGM closes the channels of communication between health services and community groups and reduces the likelihood of developing trusting relationships. The opportunity to deliver the health message is therefore lost. Health promotion is not about persuading, cajoling or coercing, or just the provision of information. It involves working with individuals and communities to make lifestyle changes by utilising a range of approaches.

The aim of health promotion for asylum-seeking women who have experienced FGM is to enhance their health potential and through health education to promote the safety of the child and other female siblings. One of the major hurdles of promoting health is to locate and engage the target population. Asylum seekers by the very nature of their trauma and temporary living accommodation can be classified as being hard to reach. If they are pregnant and not married, they may choose not to disclose the pregnancy at the induction centre because of the stigma in their native countries associated with pregnancy and marital status.

It is not uncommon for women to believe that disclosing a pregnancy negatively impacts on their asylum application. Many of these women are pregnant as a result of rape and find it extremely difficult to verbalise their experiences.[13] Equally, disclosing that they have undergone FGM is information that is private and personal to the individual and their community and is not usually readily disclosed to a stranger.

Enhancing health potential requires the woman to understand that her health could be improved. This may be very difficult, as for many years the cultural belief surrounding FGM and the torturous experience women go through has been normalised and accepted as a cultural norm and custom within their native society. In addition, asylum seekers frequently see their health as deteriorating since arriving in the host country and may therefore not believe that their health can improve. Developing a trusting relationship and delivering health education that is tailored to meet individual needs is important in order to engage with women in this situation.

The client-centred approach

The client-centred approach is a health promotion approach frequently adopted by health and social care providers and involves an equal partnership between the health professional and the woman. The woman sets the agenda and the health professionals' role is facilitative, guiding, supporting and encouraging the woman to make informed choices. The aim is facilitating the autonomy of the woman.[14] This approach makes several assumptions about the woman's role in this relationship. First, it assumes that the health professional and the woman believe that they are in partnership and indeed equal; second, it assumes that the woman will know the agenda; and third, it assumes that the woman wants autonomy.

Care providers need to be selective about the health promotion approach used. Women who are seeking asylum are not a homogenous group and have individual needs. Being asked to make a decision about an aspect of their clinical care sometimes bemuses asylum seekers. Educating women about the drive in Western culture to encourage women to be a part of decision making is important. Midwives and other health professionals should be patient with women, as this approach to healthcare may be alien to many groups. It is important to give women time to understand the different approaches to healthcare and not assume that choice is only for those who are socio-economically advantaged.

The self-empowerment approach

The process of self-empowerment involves people identifying their personal concerns, strengths, experiences and skills and utilising them to increase personal control over their own lives.[8] This approach is difficult to apply when many asylum seekers feel powerless and do not feel in control over their own lives. The decision for them to stay in the country is in the hands of the Home Office, the dispersal area is not negotiated but the decision is made on their behalf. In the induction centres they have no control over the type of food they eat or when they may like to eat and they have no resources to buy items they personally consider essential.

Midwives may seek to empower asylum-seeking women who have undergone FGM to consider reversal prior to labour. It is important that persuading and cajoling is not a part of this process. Focused education that communicates with the woman within the context of her living experiences is likely to be more effective. Through increased knowledge and understanding the woman may feel that she is in a position to make a decision.

The education approach

This approach is concerned with facilitating the learning process and enabling learning to take place through open dialogue and discussion.[14] Valuing life experiences and tailoring education to meet individual needs are integral to this process. This approach as mentioned above should be delivered at the level and within the context of the woman's daily living experiences.

The societal change approach

The aim of this approach is to ensure that health is easier to achieve. The focus is not on changing individuals' behaviour, but on positively influencing the health of society. Socio-economic disadvantage is acknowledged, as a determinant of ill health. The focus of this approach is at policy level, the aim of which is to bring about changes to society to make healthier lifestyle choices easier to attain. Working with religious and community leaders to change the mindset of those groups who wish to continue the custom of FGM has many benefits. Healthier lifestyle choices with such groups would be easier to attain if there was widespread community acceptance that FGM should be avoided.

The FGM Act 2003 contributes to making healthier lifestyle choices easier to attain. As previously discussed, this act of parliament makes it illegal for girls to be taken abroad to undergo FGM. Although it could be argued that the societal change approach is a top-down approach where the power base lies with the organisation, the 2003 FGM Act takes the onus of responsibility for not continuing the practice away from those mothers who are being pressured by other family members to organise FGM for the female members of the family.

Mental health

Promoting mental well-being is equally as significant as promoting physical health; the two areas of health have been described as being inextricably linked.

The oppression, persecution, conflict, harassment, fear, famine, rape, torture and imprisonment experienced by many asylum seekers has a negative effect on their mental health. Those who have experienced FGM hold an additional negative experience that may have caused many physical and psychological problems. Mental health problems that they suffer are no different to those of the indigenous people but may be reflected in different ways.

The National Service Framework for Mental Health (1999) calls for the development of culturally sensitive services and identifies refugees and asylum seekers as a particularly vulnerable group with a raised risk of suicide in the long term.[15] Depression during pregnancy has received greater attention over the last decade. Screening for antenatal depression and recognising those at risk of developing postnatal depression is an important area of antenatal care provision. Women who are thought to have antenatal depression should be referred to psychiatric services for further support. Women identified as being at risk of developing postnatal depression should be given additional support during the antenatal and perinatal period. The health visitor should be alerted to provide early support.

The National Service Framework for Mental Health acknowledges that asylum seekers may view mental health support services negatively because of their experiences of this service in their native countries. Midwives and health visitors should approach this subject with sensitivity. If women are referred to psychological services it may be important to reassure women that they will continue to be supported by maternity services and not abandoned to mental health.

Changing behaviour

Despite acts of parliament rendering FGM illegal, the practice has continued. Families have upheld cultural practices and traditions by taking their children out of the country to have the procedure performed. Legislation has not eradicated the practice of FGM in the UK. Sudan has been cited as having the highest prevalence of FGM in the world despite the practice being originally outlawed there in 1946 and again in 1974.

An essential prerequisite to eradicating the practice of FGM is the work of health professionals with communities where meaningful discussions should be established. Unfortunately, focusing on female genital mutilation as a control on female sexuality, as a rite of passage, as being influenced by psychosexual, sociological, mythical and religious factors, not only misrepresents the situation but is unlikely to enable health professionals to deliver an efficient health promotion service.

Further action in terms of challenging attitudes and beliefs and working with communities, influential figureheads and religious leaders may further contribute to a change in practice. The factors that continue to drive forward the practice of FGM have been explored in more detail in Chapters 1 and 2. Those who continue to subscribe to the custom hold deep-rooted beliefs; a 'belief' has been described as what one has been told or what one discovers that has no basis in current experience or any such form of knowledge that exerts some control over thoughts, actions, perceptions and motives.[16]

A belief is based on cultural information received that has been influenced by significant others, usually without any challenge. The anthropological context of

FGM and the complexity of the challenges facing health professionals should not be underestimated. Challenging attitudes and beliefs and enhancing health education is a minor component of a very complex public health problem.

Several factors that may influence change:

- community intolerance
- behaviour becomes the exception rather than the rule to a cultural group
- the presentation of new information or evidence
- acts of parliament
- the influence of colleagues, personal friends and religious leaders
- pressure from the media or the public
- the occurrence of opportunities arising from incidents
- the cost/benefit ratio moving in favour of change.

Working with communities

Social exclusion, low income, poor mental and physical health and poor access to services are not an uncommon situation for asylum seekers. Prior to dispersal, this may be tolerated and somewhat accepted, but once settled within a community these factors continue to persist and are unacceptable. The provision of care in the community is a well-established part of the midwives' role, with good examples of midwives engaging with communities across the country.[17]

Asylum seekers frequently view 'good care' as being delivered in the hospital by a doctor, a perception held from their native countries. Education about the health services and how they are delivered may help to allay fears and anxieties and reduce mistrust. Misconceptions about receiving a second-class service because the care is centred in the community may therefore be reduced.[18]

Community-based health promotion work with this group of women goes beyond the delivery of antenatal and postnatal care. It is concerned with engaging communities that may view health services as suspicious, particularly if the health message challenges strongly held beliefs about FGM. Multi-agency working may be more beneficial when setting up a service in the community. Depending on local need, midwives may choose to set up community support groups that include antenatal and postnatal education, breastfeeding support groups and one-stop drop-in services.

The Government is committed to engaging and empowering communities toward health gain and is keen for the NHS, primary care trusts and voluntary and community organisations to encourage community involvement and ensure that action on health inequality is relevant to local need.[19] Multidisciplinary and multi-agency working is the most effective way of delivering services.

The following guide may be a useful resource when planning community initiatives:

- Establish local need.
- Engage key community leaders.
- Engage key religious leaders.
- Involve existing community organisations, including local support groups.
- Involve community and voluntary organisations in service delivery.
- Promote community networks.

- Work with communities to identify their needs, ensuring services are culturally appropriate and accessible, providing better information.
- Be familiar with the local Sure Start programmes and Neighbourhood Renewal Strategy.
- Sure Start is a major initiative to reduce childhood poverty and disadvantage. Delivering services within a Sure Start area encourages a joined-up working approach where women have the opportunity to utilise appropriate services housed within the Sure Start projects.
- The national strategy for neighbourhood renewal targets the neediest communities, seeking to improve the quality and co-ordination of local activities and services including access to them.
- Collaborate with the primary care trust (PCT) to ensure that the commissioning of healthcare for marginalised groups remains high on the healthcare agenda.

Asylum seekers pregnant as a result of rape

The Black Women's Rape Action Project estimate that at least half of all women asylum seekers are pregnant as a result of rape.[20] It is estimated that this figure is vastly higher, as many rapes are unreported. Systematic rape and other forms of sexual violence have been used as weapons of war and to instil terror.

A maternity unit in a large teaching hospital in South East London provides focused support for women who are pregnant as a result of rape. In 2003 42 women disclosed that they were in this situation. All women were seeking asylum. Their countries of origin included Congo, Nigeria, Angola, Ghana, Sierra Leone, Burundi, Uganda, Somalia, Eritrea and South Africa.[13] Out of this group, 25% had undergone female genital mutilation in their formative years. After extensive counselling and support, those who had undergone FGM were offered the opportunity to attend the African Well Woman's Clinic to discuss their experiences of FGM and the benefits of reversal. Only two women attended the clinic.

Those who declined appointments felt unable to have any further invasive procedures in the vaginal area, despite understanding the process that they would need to undergo during labour. Generally the women were very withdrawn, depressed, extremely unhappy, lonely and afraid and felt desolate. Many had been gang raped and tortured. During the third and fourth counselling sessions all women felt able to disclose their experiences in more detail.

The Rogerian counselling approach proved to be somewhat ineffective in supporting these women, as they seemed reluctant to disclose their feelings but disclosed their pain and suffering. The Rogerian approach to counselling involves counsellors restricting themselves to the role of facilitator and consciously refraining from any activity which may direct the client.[21]

Unfortunately, without prompting and some direction, the women remained silent. Women frequently complained of general aches and pains and described feeling 'bad'. They also described nightmares and flashbacks they experienced. The discussion surrounding FGM with each woman was very limited from the woman's perspective. They appeared to be more concerned with their most recent trauma.

Midwives need to be mindful that women may not only have undergone FGM but they may also be survivors of rape or sexual assault. Their behaviour during invasive procedures may be guarded, they may express a reluctance to be

Box 6.2   Checklist for women who do not have support from an FGM specialist

Antenatal

- Discuss the process of childbirth.
- Discuss the procedures that take place during all stages of labour.
- If the woman is literate, encourage note-taking in her language.
- Encourage picture drawing if this aids understanding.
- Describe the second stage of labour and the need for de-infibulation in the first stage of labour.
- Discuss the reason why re-infibulation does not take place.
- Discuss changes that she will notice post de-infibulation.
- Encourage a contact visit from the health visitor antenatally.

Postnatal

- Invite discussion about the changes she has experienced.
- Invite discussion about the newborn child and FGM if this child is female.
- Do not withdraw maternity services until the health visitor is fully engaged.
- Refer for counselling support if necessary.

NB: Rape should not be recorded unless the woman consents to this. It may be just as useful to record, 'This woman has undergone war trauma, please be mindful when carrying out any invasive procedures, keep to a minimum, avoid where possible'.

examined and may experience flashbacks. Symptoms of flashbacks of trauma can seem real again and vivid for the woman. The woman may experience sensory and motor re-enactments or may faint during the experience.[22]

The medical encounter, which combines nakedness, touching, intrusion, pain or discomfort, powerlessness and depersonalisation, often leaves women feeling humiliated, dirty and re-violated.[8] A female interpreter must be utilised for those women who do not speak English and a checklist should be recorded in the notes (*see* Box 6.2).

If the labour occurs at night, all former preparation and documentation will provide a safety platform for women who may feel terrified by the prospect of labour, particularly in the absence of the interpreter, who may be unavailable during the night. Female obstetricians and midwives are best placed to support women in this position.

Reducing the barriers of communication

Communication and counselling skills remain the single most important aspect of health promotion work. Communication at a basic level involves the passing on or

---

Box 6.3 Communication 1

Amara is a 22-year-old primigravida who is pregnant as a result of rape. Her application for asylum is currently with the Home Office. Amara is booked for maternity care at the accommodation centre by the midwife. Amara's blood test reveals that she is sickle cell trait. The midwife asks about the ethnic origin of the baby's father. Amara does not respond. The midwife repeats the question but Amara does not respond. The midwife explains the reasons why the information is required. Amara does not respond. The midwife records in the maternity handheld records that 'information about the baby's father is not forthcoming'.

How could this consultation be improved?

---

transfer of information. Good communication is accepted, as being an important and integral part of the health professionals' role, but the nature and efficiency of communication should be constantly checked and reviewed. (How could the nature of communication detailed in Box 6.3 be improved?)

Good communication is essential for successful health promotion, but it is difficult to define. It involves the provision of clear, unambiguous exchange. The receiver of the message should receive the identical message that the sender intends. A distortion of this may be the result of incongruent non-verbal behaviour, so it is important that facial expression and speech are congruent.[8]

Expressing empathy, genuineness, respect and confidentiality during consultations will help to reduce the perceived barriers between the woman and the health professional. This will also encourage the development of a trusting relationship where the woman feels able to disclose personal emotive information or may feel more able to answer questions, as opposed to an environment that is perceived as 'busy' and threatening.

Effective communication is largely determined by:

- how professionals feel about themselves, as individuals – their self-worth[11]
- how the professional views the client/how the client views the professional[20]
- the professional's knowledge base about the subject
- the language used e.g. medical terminology.

Health professionals should examine personal attitudes, prejudices and belief systems prior to delivering healthcare. A constant review of attitudes and prejudices should be encouraged, as these are less static and are subject to influence and change. Stereotypical ideas encourage communication to be influenced by subjective value judgements.[8] Health professionals should not be influenced by myth or propaganda but by fact and as such treat people with dignity, empathy and respect.

Stereotypes are ideas, values and social rules that are perpetuated by society about individuals or groups. A recent example of this is negative media reports about asylum seekers that have fuelled community intolerance in parts of the UK.

Stereotypes are therefore maintained and sustained by structures within society that are seen to hold power.[8] Distorted media messages about the overstretched health services and the health needs of asylum seekers have further fuelled public uncertainty about supporting these communities and reinforced negative ideas.

A commonly reported assertion is that the increase in the numbers of asylum seekers and refugees has stretched clinical skills, resources and strained abilities to empathise with victims of torture and destitution. Singer[4] suggests that the strain on the health service has developed as a result of 25 years of underinvestment in the NHS, amounting to £237 billion, and suggests that this is a more likely reason for overstretched services.

Communication messages can be distorted if health professionals are not aware of personal prejudices, attitudes and belief systems. In a recent study that focused on communication and informed choice in the maternity care setting, economically deprived women were observed during antenatal consultations to be relatively silent, asking few questions and receiving less information than articulate economically secure women.

In some cases midwives were found to misjudge women's ability and willingness to participate in their maternity care and, as a consequence, women were negatively labelled.[23] It is suggested that stereotypes enable us to keep control and to protect ourselves in situations where we are impoverished in terms of time and resources.[23] Challenging this behaviour is vitally important if women and their families are to receive equality of healthcare provision.

Inequality in health and healthcare provision

The Black Report[24] demonstrated major socio-economic differences in health and Sir Douglas Black was quite clear in his analysis when he suggested that the root cause of inequalities in health was poverty. The 1998 Acheson report[25] advanced recommendations to reduce inequalities in health and this was further supported by *The NHS Plan*[26] and *Tackling Health Inequalities*.[1]

Political influence is further gaining momentum, with a drive from the Government to reduce the gap in infant mortality across social groups and raise life expectancy in the most disadvantaged areas faster than elsewhere. Economically deprived people have poorer health and lower life expectancy than their wealthier counterparts.[1] Strategies to reduce inequalities include targeting specific interventions including poor health issues among ethnic minority groups and mainstreaming care packages so that all services that provide care become more responsive to the needs of disadvantaged populations.

The National Institute for Clinical Excellence (NICE) guidelines suggest that women who have experienced FGM should be identified early in the antenatal period through sensitive enquiry.[27] How, when and what people present to health professionals will be influenced partly by their culture, beliefs and experiences.

Despite policy and guidance documents, inequalities in health and healthcare provision continue to persist today and are clearly evident in maternity care. Tudor Hart first described the inverse care law in 1971,[28] as the greatest need for healthcare being associated with the poorest provision. In 30 years little has changed. It is suggested that women from poorer social backgrounds are one and a half times more likely to produce a low birth weight baby or suffer perinatal death than those from other social classes.[29]

The risk of maternal death in England and Wales is known to be higher in women born abroad compared with the indigenous population and is higher in ethnic minority women.[30,31] The National Service Framework for Children, Young People and Maternity Services (2004) highlights the need to focus services to meet the needs of vulnerable marginalised groups and sets down standards to achieve this. The provision of maternity care throughout the childbirth continuum has the potential to influence the health of the mother and baby, which has a long-term impact on the future health of the nation.

Women should have easy access to supportive, high quality maternity services, designed around their individual needs and those of their babies.[19] This standard is detailed in the National Service Framework for Children, Young People and Maternity Services (2004). The Maternity Services Sub Committee of the Health Select Committee recommends that women should not need a GP referral in order to receive maternity services. The GP service is not a gatekeeping service to access maternity services. Asylum seekers and refugees frequently experience problems registering with a GP and therefore book late for maternity care.

A recent study revealed the antenatal booking patterns of asylum seekers. Out of a sample size of 61 women, two-thirds were seen in antenatal care for the first time at 22 weeks or over and 38% of these at 30 weeks or over.[32] Women from lower socio-economic groups, including ethnic minority women, booked for maternity care after 24 weeks' gestation and had missed over four routine antenatal visits.[31]

The provision of antenatal care should be accessible to local communities and meet individual needs. The National Institute for Clinical Excellence (NICE) guidelines[27] suggest that all pregnant women should be offered evidence-based information and support to enable them to make informed decisions regarding their care. One example of this is the popular Midwives Information and Resource Service (MIDIRS) informed choice leaflets. The aim of the leaflets is to provide women and health professionals with evidence-based information on a range of subjects that can be used to reinforce discussion about care practices and also used as a trigger for asking further questions. These are considered to be an excellent resource for both the midwife and the woman, with each having their respective copy detailing many areas of maternity care provision.

Unfortunately, the evaluation of the informed choice leaflets revealed negative areas of communication, particularly to the lower social groups. Women who were economically deprived were observed being treated differently from articulate economically secure women. They were less likely to be made aware of choices available to them and were given less information than more advantaged women.[33]

Moreover, dispensing the leaflets was equated with giving information and the leaflets were sometimes observed to block or pre-empt discussion. This has been described as a practice that serves to silence women.[33] Midwives should be prepared to act as advocates for women and seek their views, even more so when they speak little or no English and may be less articulate and less able to challenge the traditional patterns of care delivery that are inappropriate to their needs. The interpreter service must be utilised and female interpreters booked for these women.

Positive action for asylum seekers

In December 2002 the Health Select Committee undertook a series of enquiries into the provision of maternity services. The recommendations include better support for pregnant asylum seekers, new mothers and their babies, and warned against detaining pregnant asylum seekers. The report recommends that accommodation centres should provide a gateway to maternity services enabling quick and easy access to antenatal care. Maternity care providers and accommodation centres should work together to ensure the 'gateway' is efficient and productive.

Around the time of dispersal it is suggested that there should be better communication between maternity and child health services. The onus of responsibility has been placed on the accommodation providers to ensure that maternity services are forewarned of the woman's arrival, where test results and notes can be forwarded. The recommendations also include the need for special consideration when dispersing pregnant women to areas that are distant from their newly established friends/support network.[3] This is a positive step forward in enhancing the healthcare of asylum seekers, but this should be supported by finance and resource allocation to ensure that the implementation of changes progresses, details of which are not evident in the report.

Box 6.4   Communication 2

Amara is now 41 weeks pregnant and the midwife explains the reasons why a cervical sweep is offered at this stage of the pregnancy. During the procedure the midwife notices that Amara is reluctant for the procedure to go ahead, but encourages her. Despite encouragement Amara is still reluctant for the procedure to go ahead. The midwife asks the following questions:

1   Do you have problems down below?
2   Were you hurt when you were little?
3   Did you have problems when you were trying to make the baby?

Amara's responses to all questions was 'No'.

How could this consultation be improved?

Conclusion

Despite legislation strengthening the illegality of the act of FGM, the practice is not eradicated. The anthropological context of FGM renders the perpetuation of the practice complex and behaviour change a challenge for health professionals. Enhancing the health potential of asylum-seeking women who have undergone FGM is not a basic process and requires resource commitment and a multi-agency, multidisciplinary approach. Health promotion can only be truly effective in this situation if the process is delivered within the context of the person's everyday life. Understanding the complexities of the lives of asylum seekers and refugees challenges the Western approach to health promotion delivery.

Inequality in health and healthcare provision reinforces the subordination and marginalisation that many women feel. It also serves to perpetuate ill health disadvantage and poverty throughout generation cycles. The Government approach to enhancing health acknowledges the benefits of joined-up working and the strength to be gained from involving communities in decision making. The humanitarian rights of women must remain high on the political agenda so that policy, strategy and practice progress the good work that has already commenced. Challenging attitudes and beliefs and enhancing health education, although extremely important, is a minor component of a very complex public health problem.

References

1   Department of Health (DoH 2003) *Tackling Health Inequalities: A programme for action.* DoH, London.
2   Amnesty International (2004) *It's in our hands, stop violence against women.* Amnesty International Publications, London.
3   Secretary of State for Health (2004) *Government response to House of Commons Health Committee reports, fourth report session 2002–03: provision of maternity services eighth report session 2002–03 inequalities in access to maternity services and ninth report session 2002–03 choice in maternity services.* DoH, London.
4   Singer R (2004) Asylum seekers: an ethical response to their plight. *Lancet.* **363**: 1904.
5   British Medical Association (2002) *Asylum Seekers: meeting their healthcare needs.* British Medical Association, London, pp. 7–8.
6   Burnett A and Fassil Y (2002) *Meeting the needs of refugees and asylum seekers in the UK: an information and resource pack for health workers.* DoH, London.
7   Royal College of Midwives (RCM) (2003) *A better start: providing appropriate maternity services to refugees and asylum seekers.* RCM, London.
8   Dunkley J (2000) *Health Promotion in Midwifery Practice.* Baillière Tindall, London.
9   Maslow A (1954) *Motivation and Personality* (2e). Harper & Row, New York.
10 Crawley H (1997) *Women as Asylum Seekers: A Legal Handbook.* Immigration Law Practitioners' Association and Refugee Action, London, p. 71.
11 Department of Health (DoH 1999) *Working Together to Safeguard Children: a guide to interagency working to safeguard and promote the welfare of children.* DoH, London.
12 Department for Education and Skills (DfES 2003) *Female Genital Mutilation Act* (LASSL 2004) 4. DoH, London.
13 Dunkley-Bent J (2004) A consultant midwife's community clinic. *British Journal of Midwifery.* **12**(3): 144–71.
14 Ewles L and Simnett I (1999) *Promoting Health: a practical guide* (4e). Baillière Tindall, Edinburgh.
15 Department of Health (DoH 1999) *National Service Framework for Mental Health Modern Standards and Service Models.* DoH, London.
16 Claxton G (1988) *Live and Learn, an introduction to the psychology of growth and change in everyday life.* Open University Press, Milton Keynes.
17 Department of Health (DoH 2003) *Delivering the best midwives contribution to the NHS Plan.* Available at: www.doh.gov.uk/deliveringthenhsplan.
18 McLiesh J (2002) Mothers in exile: maternity experiences of asylum seekers in England. *Maternity Action.* **90**: 2–3.
19 Department of Health (DoH 2004) *National Service Framework for Children.* Department for Education and Skills (DfES), London.
20 Cowen T (2001) *Unequal Treatment: Findings from a refugee health survey in Barnet.* Refugee Health Access Project, London.

21 Rogers C (1974) *On Becoming A Person.* Constable, London.

22 Joseph S, Williams R and Yule W (1998) *Understanding Post-traumatic Stress: a psychological perspective on PTSD and treatment.* John Wiley & Sons Ltd., England

23 Kirkham M, Stapleton H, Thomas G and Curtis P (2002) Stereotyping as a professional defence mechanism. *British Journal Midwifery.* **10**(9): 549–52.

24 Black D, Morris JN, Smith C and Townsend P (1980) *Inequalities in Health: the Black report.* Penguin, Harmondsworth (first published by the DHSS, 1980. New introduction by P Townsend and N Davidson).

25 Acheson D (1998) *Independent Inquiry into Inequalities in Health.* The Stationery Office, London.

26 Department of Health (DoH 2000) *The NHS Plan: a plan for investment, a plan for reform.* DoH, London.

27 National Collaborating Centre for Women and Children's Health (2003) *Antenatal care, routine care for the health of pregnant women.* National Institute for Clinical Excellence, London.

28 Hart T (1971) The inverse care law. *Lancet* **1**: 405–12.

29 Donaldson LJ and Donaldson RJ (2000) *Essential Public Health* (2e). Academic Press, Newbury.

30 Ibison J, Swerdlow A, Whitehead J and Marmot M (1996) Maternal mortality in England and Wales: an analysis by country of birth. *BJOG.* **103**: 973–80.

31 Royal College of Obstetricians and Gynaecologists (RCOG 2004) *Why mothers die. Confidential inquiry into maternal and child health: improving the health of mothers, babies and children 2000–2002.* RCOG, London.

32 Kennedy P and Murphy-Lawless J (2001) *The Maternity Care Needs of Refugee and Asylum Seeking Women.* Women's Health Unit, Eastern Region Health Authority.

33 Stapleton H, Kirkham M, Curtis P and Thomas G (2002) Framing information in antenatal care. *British Journal of Midwifery.* **10**(4): 197–201.

Chapter Seven

Female genital mutilation and child protection

Adwoa Kwateng-Kluvitse

This chapter examines female genital mutilation (FGM) from the perspective of a human rights abuse and in the context of a child abuse and, therefore, a child protection issue. The chapter also highlights some of the dilemmas facing professionals working to protect girls, which may impact on their ability to carry out their duties effectively.

Cultural relativism

One issue that needs to be considered first is the idea of the universality of human rights versus the concept that human rights are culturally relative. This is a complex issue, which directly impacts women and girls, in that if one accepts that human rights are not universal then it follows that the identification, promotion and protection of human rights would be subject to State discretion rather than international legal imperative. This would then result in states placing their own traditions and cultural practices above international standards. The outcome would be detrimental to those not holding power or having status.

Despite the gains made in some developed countries, the position and power that women have in these countries is still less than that of their male counterparts. This disparity is even more pronounced in developing countries where there is a huge gulf between the status of women as compared to men. There are countries where women do not and cannot own land in their own right, where girls and women cannot choose who they will marry, where girls and women have no say in their sexual and reproductive health and rights, for example.

If human rights were culturally relative, then in countries like those described above, women and girls would be denied their human rights. Yet there are some inalienable human rights that transcend cultural and or traditional practices and it is the view of the author that no culture can legitimately practise FGM. FGM cannot be considered legitimate, legal or part of a cultural legacy, entitled to protection in any way.

FGM, like many other violations against girls and women, can clearly be identified as a human rights violation in many international instruments either by the spirit or letter of such instruments. And although many countries have signed up to these instruments, they have failed to fulfil their obligations specifically in respect of FGM. Although the 1948 Universal Declaration of Human Rights[1] did not specifically mention FGM, the statement

> Everyone has the right to a standard of living adequate for health and
> well-being of himself and his family
>
> Universal Declaration Article 25

obviously impinges on FGM. Girls and women with certain types of FGM, or who
have poor health outcomes, as a result of how FGM is performed, have been
denied the right to enjoy good health and this Declaration could have been interpreted positively and used by governments to support actions and interventions
against FGM.

In the 1979 Convention on the Elimination of All Forms of Discrimination
Against Women (CEDAW)[2] States Parties undertook

> To take all appropriate measures to modify and or abolish existing
> laws, regulations, customs and practices, which constitute discrimina-
> tion against women.
>
> CEDAW Article 2(f)

The Convention goes on to state that States Parties shall take all appropriate
measures to

> Modify the social and cultural patterns of conduct with the view of
> achieving the elimination of prejudices and customary and all other
> practices, which are based on the idea of the inferiority/superiority of
> the sexes or on stereotyped roles for men and women.
>
> CEDAW Article 5(a)

FGM is undoubtedly a cultural practice, which constitutes a discrimination against
girls and women. The Convention on the Rights of the Child (1989)[3] enshrines the
right to equality irrespective of gender/sex; it also guarantees freedom from all
forms of mental and physical violence, freedom from torture, cruel, inhuman and
degrading treatment. All States Parties are expected

> To take all effective and appropriate measures with a view to
> abolishing traditional practices prejudicial to the health of children.
>
> Convention on the Rights of the Child, Article 24(3)

As has been proven in countless studies, FGM is a hazardous practice upon health.
In 1995, in Beijing, The 'Platform for Action'[4] was unequivocal in its determination

> To ensure the full enjoyment by women and the girl child of all human
> rights and fundamental freedoms and [to] take effective action against
> violations of these rights and freedoms.
>
> The Beijing Platform for Action Paragraph 23

FGM was specifically described in the conference declaration in paragraph 41, as a
form of gender violence and as posing a grave risk to health. Governments,
international organisations and non-governmental organisations were urged to

develop policies and programmes to eliminate all forms of discrimination against the girl child – including FGM. All these instruments made it clear in the international arena that practices that perpetuate violence against girls (of which FGM is an irrefutable example) were unacceptable and action had to be taken against them.

On the African scene, African governments are also making statements against gender violence, including FGM. In the 1979 Declaration on the Rights and Welfare of the African Child[5] it was clearly recognised that there was the need to take appropriate

> Actions aimed at guaranteeing the rights and promoting the welfare of the child
> > Declaration on the Rights and Welfare of the African Child,
> > Paragraph 3

by thoroughly examining

> Cultural legacies and practices that are harmful to normal growth and development of the child; such as child marriage and female circumcision, and [that member States] should take legal and educational measures to abolish them.
> > Declaration on the Rights and Welfare of the African Child,
> > Article 3

The African Charter on Human and Peoples' Rights in 1981[6] proclaimed and agreed that everyone is entitled to

> All the rights and freedoms recognised and guaranteed in the present Charter, without distinction of any kind such as race, ethnic group, colour, sex, language ...
> > African Charter on Human and Peoples' Rights, Article 2

Article 18 of the Charter called on all States Parties to

> Ensure the elimination of every discrimination against women and also to ensure the protection of the rights of women and the child, as stipulated in international declarations and conventions.
> > African Charter on Human and Peoples' Rights, Article 18(3)

The African Charter on the Rights and Welfare of the Child (1990)[7] added to the above and recognised the paramouncy of human rights of the child and in Article 16 required States Parties to the Charter to

> Take specific legislative, administrative, social and educational measures to protect the child from all forms of torture, inhuman or degrading treatment and especially physical or mental injury of abuse, neglect or maltreatment including sexual abuse ...
> > African Charter on the Rights and Welfare of the Child, Article 16

This was further expanded in Article 21, which focused on the need to take all

> Appropriate measures to eliminate harmful social and cultural practises affecting the welfare, dignity, normal growth and development of the child and in particular; (a) those customs and practices prejudicial to the health or life of the child ...
>> African Charter on the Rights and Welfare of the Child,
>> Article 21

The 2003 Protocol to the African Charter on Human and Peoples' Rights on the Rights of Women in Africa[8] develops even further the rights and protections of women and girls by stating categorically its concern that despite States Parties ratifying the African Charter on Human and Peoples' Rights and stating their solemn commitment to eliminate all forms of discrimination and harmful practices against women, women in Africa still continue to be victims of discrimination and harmful practices.

The Protocol requires States Parties to

> Adopt and implement appropriate measures to ensure the protection of every woman's right to respect for her dignity and protection of women from all forms of violence particularly sexual and verbal violence.
>> Protocol to the African Charter on Human and Peoples' Rights
>> on the Rights of Women in Africa, Article 3(4)

Article 5 of the document focuses specifically on harmful practices, and

> Requires States Parties to prohibit and condemn all forms of harmful practices which negatively affect the human rights of women and, which are contrary to recognised international standards.
>> Protocol to the African Charter on Human and Peoples'
>> Rights on the Rights of Women in Africa, Article 5

And requires Parties to take all necessary legislative measures backed by sanctions to prohibit

> All forms of female genital mutilation, scarification, medicalisation and para-medicalisation of female genital mutilation and all other practices in order to eradicate them.
>> Protocol to the African Charter on Human and Peoples'
>> Rights on the Rights of Women in Africa, Article 5(b)

From the above it can be seen that there is a move across the world, including in Africa, to categorise FGM as an unacceptable cultural practice and there is a commitment (on paper anyway) to fight for the abandonment of the practice. The reality of the commitment of governments will be seen in the actions they support on the ground.

There have been unquestionable developments in the campaign against FGM in some African countries; there are countries that have already passed and implemented laws against FGM. Countries like Burkina Faso, Kenya, Ghana, Ivory Coast, Togo, Benin, Niger, Tanzania, Senegal, Djibouti, Chad and the Central African Republic have passed specific anti-FGM laws. In Kenya there have been successful child protection interventions using the legislation, which has protected girls from FGM while enabling them to remain at home with their parents. In Ghana, Burkina Faso, Senegal and Sierra Leone there have been reports of arrests and prosecutions in respect of instances of FGM (www.crip.org).

While legislation is critical, there is also a need to work with the communities that practise FGM to explain the need for the law and to empower parents [who are after all the primary agents of child protection] to protect their daughters from this particular form of abuse, otherwise the communities will feel under attack and the practice will only be driven underground. These positive developments point the way towards a continent in which girls [and women] will be protected from FGM.

The UK situation

Female genital mutilation first came to public notice in the early 1970s when women from the Horn of Africa fleeing civil war came to seek refuge in the UK. When these women came into contact with the National Health Service (NHS) during pregnancy and labour, FGM became apparent to service providers. Initially, because of a lack of knowledge about FGM, specifically Type 3 FGM, doctors performed Caesarean sections, as they thought that the resultant scar tissue of FGM was a congenital abnormality.

These medical interventions were an anathema to the women; firstly because of the widely held cultural view that women should deliver vaginally, and secondly, because inevitably they became objects of curiosity in the hospitals. Women were very unhappy with the services they were receiving from the NHS, but did not know where and how to complain to improve services.

In 1980, the Minority Rights Group published a document entitled *Female Circumcision, Excision and Infibulation*,[9] which examined the practice of FGM. This was followed by a further publication entitled *Female Genital Mutilation: proposals for change*.[10] Although neither of these publications caused a huge reaction among the general populace, they did lead to women activists getting together to form a non-governmental organisation (NGO) dedicated to a campaign against FGM.

The Prohibition of Female Circumcision Act 1985

The legislative campaign against FGM started in the early 1980s, headed by small NGOs and a few dedicated politicians who fought to get the first legislation against FGM passed. In 1982, activists and parliamentarians campaigned for legislation against FGM. The first time an FGM bill was presented to Parliament in 1982, it met with a great deal of opposition from the ruling Conservative Party, which instituted a three-line whip, which resulted in that Bill being defeated.

The Government disagreed with the Bill on the grounds that they felt it would alienate minority groups and that that any action taken against these African refugee communities would be construed as racist, and that the numbers affected by FGM were unknown. Their concern was not about the fact FGM constituted an abuse. Later on, the Government itself introduced a very similar Bill, which resulted in the 1985 Prohibition of Female Circumcision Act[11] (PFCA) being passed, making the performance of FGM in England, Ireland and Wales illegal and putting FGM squarely in the child protection arena. The law made it illegal for anyone to

> Excise, infibulate or otherwise mutilate the whole or any part of the labia majora or minora or clitoris of another person or to aid abet, counsel or procure the performance by another person of any of those acts on that other person's own body'.
> Prohibition of Female Circumcision Act 1985 Para I (a)

The penalty for flouting the law was a fine of £1000 or a term of imprisonment not exceeding 6 months or both. This law provided a framework on which to develop other child protection initiatives.

The Children Act 1989

In 1989, the Government passed a new law on the protection of children. The Children Act[12] was an attempt to codify existing laws into one comprehensive law. Although the Children Act did not specifically mention FGM, because FGM is clearly an abuse of children it is covered by the Act.

In 1999, the Department of Health (DoH) produced *Working Together to Safeguard Children*,[13] a document intended to set out guidelines on how all agencies and professionals should work together to promote children's welfare and protect them from abuse and neglect. The guidelines were intended to provide a structure within which local authorities were to deal with issues of child protection.

FGM is specifically mentioned in the chapter entitled 'Child Protection in Specific Circumstances'. The chapter states that local authorities may exercise their powers under Section 47 of the Children Act if they believe that a child is likely to be/has been the subject of FGM. It also states that local authorities should be alert to the possibility of FGM among the ethnic communities, and should focus on a preventative strategy involving community education if they are aware of numbers of practising communities in their area.

Female Genital Mutilation Act 2003

Subsequent to the PFCA being enacted, it soon became clear to the NGOs working in the field that communities were circumventing the existing legislation by taking their daughters home 'on holiday' and having FGM performed there. This gap in the law resulted in girls not being fully protected from FGM and the campaign to have the law amended started.

In 2003, a private members bill supported by the Government was legislated. (Although the legislation was signed into law in Oct 2003, it was not enacted until March 2004.) The amended law is called the Female Genital Mutilation Act 2003.[14] The most significant development in this piece of legislation is the introduction of the concept of 'extra-territoriality'. With the introduction of extra-territoriality, girls who are UK nationals or UK permanent residents cannot be removed from the UK for purposes of FGM and returned to England without parents being prosecuted for the offence of 'aiding, abetting, counselling or procuring a girl to excise, infibulate or otherwise mutilate the whole or any part of her labia majora, labia minora or clitoris' (FGM Act 2003, Paragraph 2).

This protection applies irrespective of the legislation in the country to which the girl was removed. The UK Government intends this 2003 law to strengthen and reinforce the provisions of the 1985 Act. In theory therefore, girls from practising communities should be protected from FGM anywhere in the United Kingdom and UK nationals/permanent residents should be protected from FGM anywhere in the world.

The FGM Act 2003 currently only applies to England, Wales and Northern Ireland. The Scottish Parliament is currently reviewing the legislation in relation to Scotland.

The legislation against FGM is reinforced by child protection procedures. All Social Service Departments must adhere to such procedures to ensure the protection of children at risk of harm. Risk of FGM is clearly a risk of significant harm. In 2003, the London Child Protection Procedures came into effect for all Social Service Departments in London. It was thought important to standardise child protection procedures in an effort to improve services to all.

The authorities have deemed it necessary to develop these pan-London procedures for two reasons: firstly, because of the fact that all the different local authorities have different policies and procedures in relation to child protection, and secondly, because several inquiries into the deaths of children known to the statutory sector have consistently highlighted the same issues of concern, including issues around the lack of communication between agencies and individuals, failure of professionals to follow child protection guidance and issues relating to highly mobile families.

The guidelines of the London Child Protection Procedures[15] reaffirm the philosophy of the Children Act 1989. The first principle is the 'paramouncy principle' i.e. the welfare of the child is paramount and overrides all other considerations when a child is at risk. Other principles include: intervention when a child has suffered or is at risk of suffering significant harm; the need to work in partnership with other agencies, parents and carers; the 'no-order principle' i.e. that court orders will be made only when necessary (cases should be resolved with the minimum of court intervention); and the wishes and feelings of the child should be ascertained and considered (if the child/ren are of an age and understanding).

The London Child Protection Procedures deal with FGM as a specific issue with set timescales and standards to assist social workers to complete their task. The procedures state that FGM must always be regarded as causing significant harm and the first strategy meeting must be held within two days if there is a suspicion of threatened or actual FGM.

The second meeting must take place within 10 working days of the referral with the aim of preventing the girl from going through FGM or supporting her if she has already undergone FGM. The procedures indicate that the main emphasis of the work should be though 'education and persuasion' which should be reflected in the child protection plan, but there is an admonition to ensure that the Police Child Protection Unit be informed at the earliest point in the event that there would be a criminal investigation (*see* Figure 7.1).

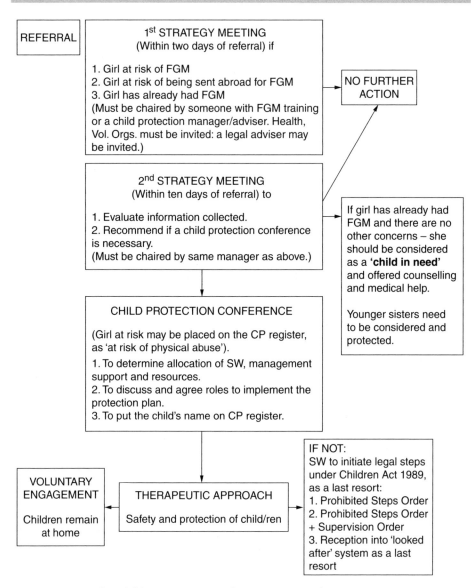

Figure 7.1 London child protection procedures in respect of FGM

It must be noted that child protection procedures existed prior to the introduction of the London Procedures. However, they were individually developed by Local Authority Social Service Departments and later by Area Child Protection Committees. As a result, different local authorities developed many different procedures for actual or suspected FGM. Some departments classified FGM as a category of child sexual abuse and responded using those standards, while others classified it as a form of physical abuse and therefore responded according to those timescales. Still others developed unique and separate procedures for social workers to follow in response to FGM.

Despite these differences in classification there have been several child protection interventions at local level, which have succeeded in protecting girls. With the introduction of the new legislation, there is an additional element of protection, although the differences in procedures will continue to exist outside London for some time.

Dilemmas

On paper and in theory, the child protection polices and procedures in respect of FGM are fairly clear. There are still, unfortunately, cases where the procedures fail to protect girls at risk. There are several reasons for these failures and FORWARD's experiences suggest the following obstacles to zero tolerance of the practice of FGM.

Legal and moral responsibility

While for professionals their responsibilities in respect of child protection are clearly codified, the same standards do not apply to members of the public. While there is an exhortation that members of the public who are aware of children at risk (of any abuse) should report it to the authorities, there is no legal requirement that they do so, neither do they face a legal penalty if they do not do so. This can therefore result in a situation where members of the public may be aware that a girl is at risk but fail to report it.

Personal dilemmas

Policies and procedures on paper do not reflect the very real dilemmas social workers face in responding to cases of actual or suspected FGM. There are still not enough social workers from FGM-practising communities who have the expertise and ability to work with families where FGM is an issue. It is also unfair to assume/expect that just because workers are from FGM-practising communities they are willing or (indeed) able to deal with FGM.

Women who have undergone FGM but have not yet been able to internally resolve the issue will be under a great deal of psychological stress and distress if they are faced with 'working a case' as part of their workload without specific support tailored to their life experiences. On the other hand, there is the extreme reaction of workers from non-FGM practising communities who respond to what they perceive as a totally 'barbaric practice' with emotion and with a judgemental attitude. Such workers are unable to put their Eurocentric views to one side temporarily to work the case in a sensitive manner, and overreact.

There is also the response of workers who, not knowing enough about FGM, are confused by the labels of culture, tradition and religion which are raised whenever FGM is mentioned. Such workers end up not taking any action at all, because they are aware that in most cases these girls are very much loved and because parents sincerely believe that they are doing what is in the long-term best interests of their daughters.

All these responses are inappropriate, unhelpful and fail to protect the girl and her siblings from harm. The response needed from the statutory sector must be a considered and well-thought-out one, which is implemented calmly, while being cognisant of the socio-cultural context in which FGM occurs.

In some cases women from FGM-practising communities may be unaware of the health consequences, the legislative framework and the human rights violations inherent in FGM. They may be personally against FGM but unable to withstand the societal pressure to conform; they may not, because of the traditions of their community, have the power to make any decisions about anything to do with raising their children (all that power may be vested in her in-laws); she may not even know that she has any other option apart from to subject her daughters to the knife. Such women can be worked with and they can be empowered to protect their daughters.

However, there will be some women who are adamant and insist on performing FGM, irrespective of any information or support they are given. The key task of statutory sector workers is to ensure that girls are protected from any form of FGM and to use any remedies available to them to ensure the paramouncy principle.

Recommendations

It is the author's sincere belief that it is possible for practising communities to abandon FGM, but that this process must be assisted by the statutory sector in the UK. The following recommendations would go some way to facilitate communities' change of attitude and behaviour while ensuring that girls are protected from this form of abuse.

1   In order to ensure that all girls at risk are protected from FGM it is imperative that all members of the statutory sector are aware of the issues surrounding FGM, the risk factors and what their personal roles and responsibilities are in the event of actual or suspected cases of FGM. All staff should have some basic training in FGM. For those who are likely to encounter it in the course of their duties, FGM should be a compulsory module in the core curricula and should not only deal with practice issues but also with the conflicting emotions that FGM arouses.

2   It is also important that all members of the statutory sector are approaching FGM from the same standpoint, so that the information being provided to practising communities is the same. This is particularly critical to prevent any muddled messages being received by communities. For people for whom FGM is the norm, who may be struggling internally with the culture conflict they are enduring, mixed messages will result in them falling into old ways of thinking and behaving, and FGM being perpetuated.

3   In terms of preventative work, it would be a positive innovative initiative for local authorities/primary care trusts who are aware that they have significant numbers of practising communities in their boroughs to undertake preventative education programmes with those communities. One way of doing this would be to tie grant aid to activities against FGM, as well as undertaking some of the activities themselves. Days like International Women's Day and the International Day of Violence Against Women could be used to discuss issues of women's health and rights including FGM.

4   For children to be able to identify the risk they may face from FGM and other types of abuse, FGM should be dealt with in the school setting, in much the

same way that children are taught about sexual and physical abuse and what to do in the event that they are exposed to any of them. The only caveat is that the teachers who are dealing with the topic must be very conversant and comfortable with the topic and must be able to put it in the context of other abuses of children without children being the butt of ridicule and ostracism in the playground.

5   Health services must be geared up to respond to the needs of women who have undergone FGM. These services must be culturally appropriate and sensitive and should also perform an educative and empowering function. Too often, the health aspects are resolved but there is little opportunity taken to undertake further educative work with the woman and her partner.

In conclusion, FGM is a deeply entrenched cultural practice that has long-term effects on the lives of women and girls. It is important that the UK have a considered systematic response to it, as there are significant numbers of women affected and girls at risk now living in the UK. Legislation, policy and practice must all work together so that future generations of girls can grow up in a world without female genital mutilation.

References

1   General Assembly of the United Nations (1948) *Universal Declaration of Human Rights.* United Nations General Assembly, New York.

2   General Assembly of the United Nations (1979) *Convention on the Elimination of All Forms of Discrimination Against Women.* United Nations General Assembly, New York.

3   General Assembly of the United Nations (1989) *The Convention on the Rights of the Child.* United Nations General Assembly, New York.

4   United Nations (1995) *Beijing Declaration and Platform for Action.* Fourth World Conference on Women, Beijing.

5   United Nations (1979) *Declaration on the Rights and Welfare of the African Child* (AHG/ ST. 4 Rev. 1) adopted by the Assembly of Heads of State and Government of the Organization of African Unity, at its Sixteenth Ordinary Session in Monrovia, Liberia, 17–20 July.

6   Organisation of African Unity (OAU) (1981) *African Charter on Human and Peoples' Rights.* Organisation of African Unity, Addis Ababa.

7   Organisation of African Unity (OAU) (1990) *African Charter on the Rights and Welfare of the Child.* Organisation of African Unity, Addis Ababa.

8   Organisation of African Unity (OAU) (2003) *Protocol to the African Charter on Human and Peoples' Rights on the Rights of Women in Africa.* Organisation of African Unity, Addis Ababa.

9   Dorkenoo E (1980) *Female Circumcision, Excision and Infibulation.* Minority Rights Group, London.

10 Dorkenoo E and Elworthy S (1983) *Female Genital Mutilation: proposals for change.* Minority Rights Group, London.

11 HM Government (UK) (1995) *Prohibition of Female Circumcision Act.* Her Majesty's Stationery Office, London.

12 HM Government (UK) (1989) *Children Act.* Her Majesty's Stationery Office, London.

13 Department of Health (DoH) (1999) *Working Together to Safeguard Children.* Department of Health, London.

14 HM Government (UK) (2003) *Female Genital Mutilation Act.* The Stationery Office, London.

15 London Child Protection Committee (2003) *London Child Protection Procedures.* lcpc@alg. gov.uk, London.

Chapter Eight

Strategies for FGM prevention in Europe

Els Leye

Introduction

This chapter offers a brief review of how the problem of FGM is being dealt with in Europe. The first section gives an estimate of the magnitude of the problem of FGM in Europe, including a definition of the critical problems in assessing the prevalence of FGM in Europe. This is followed by an account of the various strategies used in Europe to handle FGM, including policy and legislative issues, education and prevention initiatives, a brief overview of the initiatives taken by the health sector and some research priorities on FGM in Europe. In conclusion, recommendations are presented for effective strategies for the prevention of FGM in Europe.

Prevalence of female genital mutilation in Europe

To date, there is no actual data available on the practice of FGM in Europe, either on the total number of women and girls that have undergone the practice, or on the number of girls that might be at risk. However, establishing the magnitude of the problem of FGM in Europe is paramount in order to substantiate the claim for funds and to measure changes in behaviour,[1] as well as to monitor the increase or decrease of the number of women with FGM and girls at risk.[2]

Anecdotal evidence exists of the prevalence in some European countries, and can be retrieved from literature. In France, 4500 girls are estimated to be at risk of FGM, and estimations of women with FGM vary from 13 000 to 30 000.[3,4] Approximately 21 000 women with FGM live in Germany and an estimated 5500 girls might be at risk.[5] Data from the Ministry of Interior of 1994 estimates that 28 000[6] women with FGM live in Italy, while there are at least 4000 to 5000 girls with FGM in the country.[7] Jäger et al. estimate that there were approximately 6700 girls at risk of FGM and women who have undergone the procedure in Switzerland.[8] 86 000 first generation immigrant refugees/asylum-seeking women and girls who have undergone FGM live in the UK.[9]

Another way of establishing the magnitude of the problem is estimating the number of women with, and the number of girls at risk of, FGM, based on census data and by extrapolation from country of origin prevalence data. This method gives an indication of the scale of the problem in Europe, but it is important to note that it also meets several critical problems:[10,11,12]

- The estimations are based on census data, and this census data is based on nationality of women (country of birth or citizenship), but does not take into account the ethnic groups to which these women belong, although ethnicity or the region where women come from would give a much more accurate picture of the presence of FGM than nationality.
- Country of origin prevalence data is often imprecise because it too is based upon estimates ranging from 'most reliable' to 'questionable' estimates.[13]
- Estimations derived from census data do not take into account asylum seekers and illegal women. However, asylum applications need to be taken into account in order to assess the effect that including asylum seekers might have on the actual number of the population affected by FGM in each Western country. Methods of reaching illegal people should be examined in order to take this population into account.
- Second generation immigrants are difficult to trace; girls of this category might still be at risk of FGM.
- Census data is not flexible enough to take into account migration flows that influence the foreign population of a country.
- Comparisons between countries are problematic. Variations exist between the main sources of information on migration, across countries, which makes comparison of figures difficult, if not impossible.

In the framework of research on current legal provisions in Europe with regard to FGM,[1] estimations were calculated for Belgium, Spain, Sweden and the UK that are included in the boxes below. The data on Italy are derived from a research report of Nosotras, an Italian NGO based in Firenze.[14]

Belgium[15]

Based on census data of 1 January 2002, the total number of female foreigners in Belgium from African FGM risk countries is estimated at 12 415, asylum seekers and illegal migrants not included. Based on the extrapolation of country of origin prevalence data, the share of women with FGM in this population is estimated at 2745. In this group, a total of 534 girls are from African countries where FGM is practised and are in the age group at risk of FGM (0–14 years). Most of these women/girls are from Ghana (30% prevalence) and the Democratic Republic of Congo (5% prevalence).

Spain[16]

About 3000 migrant girls younger than 16 years come from countries where FGM is practised (census 2001). Most of the women/girls come from Senegal (20% prevalence), the Gambia (80% prevalence) and Ghana. The Gambian girls are the major risk group, both due to their number (1265 girls younger than 16 years in November 2001) and to the prevalence of FGM in their country of origin.

Sweden[17]

In Sweden, the largest groups of Africans from an FGM-practising country are Somalis (98% prevalence), followed by Ethiopians (80% prevalence). Based on census data of 2002, 1138 Somali and 308 Ethiopian girls are in the age group at risk of FGM (0–15 years). Somalis live primarily in Sweden's three biggest cities, i.e. Stockholm, Gothenburg and Malmö.

United Kingdom[18]

Estimating the prevalence for the UK has to deal with a particular problem: census information does not categorise communities by country of origin and thus it is impossible to ascertain the numbers of practising communities living in the UK. Based on statistics from the 1999 Labour Force Survey (only six African risk countries are included and only those immigrants that outnumber 6000 are included in this survey), the extrapolation indicates that possibly 5444 girls under 16 years might be at risk of FGM and 69 875 women are already affected. Further extrapolation including the remaining countries known to practise FGM gives an estimation of 22 000 girls at risk and 279 500 women already affected. Most of the women at risk come from Kenya (38% prevalence), Somalia and Egypt (97% prevalence).

Italy[14]

The estimated number of women with FGM in Italy, based on census data from 2000, is 32 881. Most of these women come from Somalia (7422), Nigeria (5966, 25% prevalence in country of origin), Egypt (5266) and Ethiopia (4180).

Strategies for FGM prevention in Europe

FGM on the international and European agenda

The box below provides a non-exhaustive list of international texts and resolutions (binding and non-binding) in which FGM is directly condemned or which can be used as a basis to reject FGM. To have an overview of countries that ratified these international covenants, conventions, declarations, etc. and to read more about these texts, I refer to the literature (see, for example, Leye *et al.* (2004), Rahman *et al.* (2000), Smith (1995)[1,19,20]).

- The Universal Declaration on Human Rights (adopted 1948)
- The European Convention for the Protection of Human Rights and Fundamental Freedoms (adopted 1955)

- The International Covenant on Civil and Political Rights (adopted 1966)
- The International Covenant on Economic, Social and Cultural Rights (adopted 1966)
- The International Convention on the Elimination of All Forms of Discrimination Against Women (adopted 1979)
- 'Banjul Charter': African Charter on Human Rights and Peoples' Rights (adopted 1981)
- The Convention of the Rights of the Child (adopted 1989)
- Recommendation no 19 of the UN Committee on the Elimination of Discrimination Against Women (adopted 1992)
- Vienna Declaration and Action Programme adopted at the World Conference on Human Rights (held in 1993)
- Declaration of UN General Assembly on the Elimination of Violence against Women (adopted 1993)
- Declaration and Action Programme of the UN Conference on Population and Development (Cairo, 1994)
- Declaration and Action Programme of the Fourth World Conference on Women (Beijing, 1995)
- African Charter on the Rights and Welfare of the Child (Banjul, 1998).
- Additional Protocol to the African Charter on Human and Peoples' Rights on the Rights of Women (Maputo, 2003)
- Cairo Declaration on the Elimination of FGM (Cairo, 2003).

Interest in FGM at the European Union (EU) policy level is increasing steadily, but as yet general strategies applicable in all Member States are not available.[12,21] Some of the important steps forward can be listed as follows:

A First Study Conference on FGM in Europe was held in London (UK) in July 1992 and organised by the Foundation for Women's Health Research and Development (FORWARD). The conference was called to respond to the need for action against the practice of FGM in Europe and other Western countries. The conference aimed at developing a co-ordinated, unified approach to the abolition of the practice in Europe and other Western countries (London Declaration, 6–8 July 1992).

A Second Study Conference on FGM in Europe was held in Gothenburg (Sweden) in July 1998. The conference was organised by the Committee of the Regions of the European Union and the City of Gothenburg, with the technical co-operation of WHO, Geneva. The conference came up with recommendations for an Action Plan for Europe (Gothenburg Declaration, 1–3 July 1998).

At the request of the European Commission (EC), the International Centre for Reproductive Health (ICRH) organised an expert meeting in November 1998* with experts from Africa, the USA and Europe. The goal of the expert meeting was to formulate recommendations for the development of a strategy to tackle

---

*The expert meeting was organised in Ghent, Belgium in 1998 with funds from the European Commission (Daphne) in collaboration with the Royal Tropical Institute of Amsterdam, Defence for Children International Section (the Netherlands) and with the Groupement pour l'Abolition des Mutilations Sexuelles (GAMS), Belgium.

FGM in Europe. The recommendations were submitted to the EC, together with a background paper on particularly sensitive issues and potential pitfalls associated with the various measures proposed. The recommendations focused on guidelines for three groups of professionals who deal with FGM: community outreach and social workers, healthcare professionals and the judiciary.

On 29 November 2000, an International Day Against Female Genital Mutilation was organised in the European Parliament (EP) to mobilise support for a motion for a resolution proposing (amongst other things) that EU Member States provide asylum to all women who want to escape FGM.

In Autumn 2000, the European Women's Lobby started a one year European Campaign on Women Asylum Seekers to highlight the forms of persecution that are unique to women and which require recognition in law: female genital mutilation, forced marriages, the stoning to death for presumed adultery, and guilt by association, to name but a few.

The European Network for the Prevention and Eradication of Harmful Traditional Practices Affecting the Health of Women and Children, In Particular Female Genital Mutilation (EuroNet FGM) was founded in March 2002, following ample discussions in Dakar (1997), Göteborg and Ghent (1998) and following a one year project (implemented in 2000) that aimed at establishing such a network. In this project (funded by the EC Daphne programme), priorities for future networking in Europe were discussed as well as a Charter and Statutes.[22] Founding members of the Network are from nine EU countries (Belgium, France, Denmark, Italy, UK, Germany, Spain, Sweden and the Netherlands).

The issue of FGM is also mentioned in the relations of the European Commission with developing countries. For the first time, the prevention of FGM has been explicitly mentioned in the Cotonou Agreement (June 2000).* In a Communication from the European Commission to the Council of Ministers,[†] the prevention of female genital mutilation is mentioned as one of the main objectives of international co-operation in the area of population and family planning.

In November 2000, the Women's World Forum Against Violence – in its Final Statement on Female Genital Mutilation – held in Valencia in Spain, called for intensified action to be taken immediately to speed up the elimination of FGM worldwide. The Council of Europe also decided to include a specific budget line 'Female genital mutilation' in the 2001 budget for the Daphne programme (decision of 14 December 2001) on the Prevention of Violence Against Children, Young People and Women.

At the initiative of the Swedish National Board of Health and Welfare and the Swedish NGO RISK, an expert meeting gathered at the European Parliament in Strasbourg (France) in April 2001 to develop a Joint Agenda for Preventing and Eliminating FGM, to be presented to the European Commission, European Parliament and to relevant United Nations agencies. The Agenda was developed

---

* The Cotonou Agreement replaces the Lomé Convention. Since 1975, this agreement has provided a framework for trade and co-operation between ACP (Asian, Caribbean and Pacific) countries and the European Community. The Cotonou Agreement is a 20-year partnership agreement with 77 ACP countries.

[†] Communication from the Commission to the Council on the compendium providing policy guidelines in specific areas or sectors of co-operation to be approved by the Community within the ACP-EC Council of Ministers, 5 July 2000.

drawing on declarations, recommendations and statements, and on the experiences of working towards the elimination of FGM in Africa and Europe, and was used for developing a report on FGM (by MEP Elena Valenciano – see below).

The European Parliamentary Committee on Women's Rights and Equal Opportunities developed a report on female genital mutilation (Rapporteur: Elena Valenciano Martínez-Orozco, Report no A5–0285/2001), including a resolution on FGM of the European Parliament. The Resolution on FGM was adopted by the European Parliament on 20 September 2001 (2001/2035 (INI)). Although not legally binding, the adoption of the Resolution shows the commitment of the European Parliament to act against FGM.

The EP report on Sexual and Reproductive Rights (Rapporteur: Anne Van Lancker, Report no A5–0223/2002, 6 June 2002), mentions in its motion for resolution that FGM has a damaging effect on sexual relations, pregnancies and childbirth.

On 10 and 11 December 2002, a conference was organised at the European Parliament in Brussels, to launch the Stop FGM Campaign and to make public the 'International Appeal against Female Genital Mutilation'. This campaign is a joined initiative by AIDOS, 'No Peace without Justice' and TAMWA (Tanzanian Women Association).

On 15 July 2003, the European Parliament and the Council of Europe adopted the Regulation (EC) No 1567/2003 on 'Aid for policies and actions on reproductive and sexual health and rights in developing countries'. This Regulation states that community financial support shall be given to specific operations targeting the poorest and most vulnerable populations in both rural and urban areas, and in particular to those which aim to: '[…] (d) combat practices harmful to the sexual and reproductive health of women, adolescents and children, such as female genital mutilation, sexual violence, child marriages and early marriages'.

On 19 November 2003, the EP adopted a resolution on the Violation of Women's Rights and the international relations of the EU. This resolution stresses again that FGM is an unacceptable form of violence perpetrated against women and girls, and urges Member States to pass legislation – or to ensure that existing legislation is more strictly complied with – prohibiting and imposing penalties for genital mutilation in their own country, and at the same time to develop national prevention programmes in order to ultimately eradicate the practice of genital mutilation.

Other EP resolutions that specifically mention FGM are the 'Resolution on children's rights and child soldiers in particular' (adopted by the ACP-EU Joint Parliamentary Assembly on October 2003) and the 'Resolution on poverty-related diseases and reproductive health in ACP States, in the context of the 9th EDF', that has been adopted by the ACP-EU Joint Parliamentary Assembly on 19 February 2004.

In the *Report on population and development: 10 years after the UN Conference in Cairo* (2003/2133 (INI)) (Rapporteur Karin Junker, Report no A5–0055/2004), the European Parliament calls on all governments to prohibit harmful traditions and practices, such as FGM, and to launch information campaigns on this subject in order to show that 'they constitute an unacceptable violation of the bodily integrity of women, that they are a significant threat to health and may even result in death'. This report, which evaluated the process made in achieving the goals of Cairo, was adopted in 2004.

Box 8.1   Some of the main issues with regard to FGM in Europe in the EP Resolution on Female Genital Mutilation (2001/2035(INI)):

[...] The European Parliament,

- Calls upon Member States to harmonise existing legislation;
- Opposes any form of medicalisation;
- Urges Member States to involve communities when adopting measures;
- Rejects any scientific or religious basis for justifying the practice;
- Condemns FGM as a violation of human rights;
- Calls upon the European Union and the Member States to pursue, condemn and punish the carrying out of these practices, by applying an integrated strategy, which takes into account the legislative, health and social dimensions and the integration of the immigrant population;
- Calls on the Commission to draw up a complete strategy in order to eliminate FGM in the EU, establishing legal and administrative, preventive, educational and social mechanisms to enable women who are at risk to obtain protection;
- Asks the Commission to carry out an awareness campaign directed at legislators/parliaments in the countries of origin to maximise the impact of legislation or to facilitate the formulation and adoption of such legislation;
- Calls on the Council, Commission and Member States to carry out an in-depth enquiry to ascertain the extent of FGM in the Member States;

[...]

National laws in Europe with regard to FGM[23]

Legal provisions pertaining to FGM are found in a variety of sources, including criminal laws and child protection laws. In Europe, some countries developed specific legislation on FGM; in other countries FGM is prosecutable under the general penal code and/or child protection provisions.

The following gives a review of laws regarding female genital mutilation in the former 15 EU Member States. This review is based on a research study performed on legal provisions related to FGM in these Member States, and on the difficulties of implementing these laws.*

---

*The study was financed by the European Commission (Daphne programme), ran from 1 January 2003 to 30 June 2004 and was carried out by the International Centre for Reproductive Health (Ghent University, Belgium) in partnership with the Lund University Department of Sociology (Sweden); University of Valencia, Centre of Studies on Citizenship, Migration and Minorities (Spain), Foundation for Women's Health, Research and Development (FORWARD, UK), the 'Commission pour l'Abolition des Mutilations Sexuelles' (CAMS, France) and the Centre for Human Rights (Ghent University, Belgium).

Table 8.1 Specific criminal law provisions applicable in former EU Member States[1]

	Austria	Belgium	Denmark	Spain	Sweden	United Kingdom
Specific criminal law provision	Section 90 of the Penal Code	Article 409 of the Penal Code	Articles 245–246 of the Penal Code	Article 149 of the Penal Code	Act Prohibiting Genital Mutilation of women, 1982:316, changed in 1998 and 1999	PFC Act 1985 and changed in the FGM Act in 2003
Date of entering into force	01/01/2002	27/03/2001	01/06/2003	01/10/2003	01/07/1982, modified in 1998 and 1999	1985, modified to FGM Act 2003 on 03/03/2004
Applicable on genital mutilation of boys	Yes	No	No	Yes	No	No
Which forms of FGM are forbidden?	Clitoridectomy Excision Infibulation All other forms	Clitoridectomy Excision Infibulation All other forms, except tattoos and piercings	Clitoridectomy Excision Infibulation –	Clitoridectomy Excision Infibulation All other forms	Clitoridectomy Excision Infibulation All other forms	Clitoridectomy Excision Infibulation All other forms, except tattoos, piercing and stretching of the labia
Is re-infibulation mentioned?	Not specifically stipulated as illegal	Not specifically stipulated as illegal	Not specifically stipulated as illegal, national guidelines are provided	Not specifically stipulated as illegal	Not specifically stipulated as illegal, national guidelines are provided	Not specifically stipulated as illegal, health professional guidelines are provided

Aggravating circumstances	Loss of essential body parts/Permanent and incurable corporal lesions/Permanent loss of working capacity/Offence causes death	Offence is committed against minor/Offence is performed by a parent, person having custody/Permanent and incurable corporal lesions/Permanent loss of working capacity/Offence causes death	Loss of essential body parts/Permanent and incurable corporal lesions/Offence endangers life of victim/Offence causes death	Offence is committed against a minor/Offence is performed by a parent, person having custody	Offence endangers life of the victim/The crime involved particularly reckless behaviour	Not mentioned in the 1985 Act, or in the 2003 FGM Act
Does the consent of the victim affect the legal qualification of the act?	No	No	No	No	No	No
Applicability of the principle of extraterritoriality	Yes	Yes	Yes	Yes	Yes	Not in the 1985 Act, but in the 2003 FGM Act
Criminal prosecution of FGM?	No	No	No	Yes (in these court cases FGM was still treated under general criminal law)	No	No

PFC: Prohibition of Female Circumcision

Specific criminal law provisions

In six European countries, specific criminal law provisions have been developed: Austria, Belgium, Denmark, Spain, Sweden and the United Kingdom. With the exception of Sweden and the UK, all laws have been developed very recently. In none of these countries have cases been brought to court under these specific criminal law provisions. In all six countries, the principle of extraterritoriality is applicable, which makes FGM punishable even if the offence is committed outside the frontiers of the country.

Gaps in some of the specific criminal laws were identified, more specifically with regard to the issue of male circumcision, re-infibulation, piercing and cosmetic vaginal surgery.[1]

- **Male circumcision:** the specific criminal law provisions in Austria and Spain do not clearly specify that the law is specifically related to 'female' genital mutilation. Consequently, these laws could also be applicable to male circumcision, making it technically illegal, although it is questionable if this was meant to be the case.
- **Re-infibulation:** Professionals are sometimes confronted with requests to 'close' a woman after delivery to her 'infibulated' state before delivery. Key question is: 'what is the difference between re-suturing an episiotomy and a re-infibulation, and how should professionals deal with such a question when the law is not clear about it?' The laws in these six countries have no specifications concerning the issue of re-infibulation, although in Denmark, Sweden and the UK national guidelines are provided with regard to the issue of re-infibulation.
- **Piercing:** This falls under the WHO Type 4 of FGM ('[...] type 4 includes pricking, piercing or incision of the clitoris and /or labia [...]'). Only Belgium and the UK have excluded piercing specifically from the types of FGM forbidden by their laws.
- **Cosmetic surgery:** Specific laws that have been developed are not clear about the difference between what is considered FGM and what is considered a so-called 'designer vagina', an emerging trend in Europe and the USA. Furthermore, the consent of the victim does not affect the legal qualification of the act in the countries with a specific law. For example, Swedish law does not mention age or ethnic background and considers consent irrelevant. Consequently, the Swedish Act on FGM technically outlaws genital changes in all women, and all gynaecol-
- ogists or plastic surgeons performing such alterations to the genitalia for non-medical reasons could be prosecuted. The key question here is: is the law clear that purchasing a designer vagina is prohibited for all women because it can be considered FGM, or is the law only applicable in relation to African women?

Table 8.1 gives details on the specific criminal law provisions in Austria, Belgium, Denmark, Spain, Sweden and the United Kingdom, the 6 former EU Member States with a specific law on FGM.

General criminal law provisions

In all other former European Member States (Finland, France, Germany, Greece, Ireland, Italy, Luxembourg, Portugal and the Netherlands), FGM is forbidden under general criminal law. Criminal prosecutions for FGM occurred only in France and Italy.

The criminal offence consists of (serious) bodily injury and aggravating circumstances can be taken into account, such as: the offence is committed against a minor, the offence causes death, the offence is performed by a parent/person having custody, etc. The principle of extraterritoriality is not applied in Finland, Greece, Ireland, Luxembourg and Portugal.

At the moment (November 2004), discussion is ongoing in Portugal and Ireland with regard to the inclusion of a specific criminal law provision on FGM in the Penal Code. Extraterritoriality, with the exigency of the principle of double incrimination, is applicable in the Netherlands and Germany. This makes FGM punishable when it is committed outside the frontiers of the country, but on condition that FGM is also an offence in the country where the crime was committed. In the Netherlands and Germany, another condition to this principle is that the offender must have Dutch or German nationality. The Netherlands are, however, discussing the removal of the principle of double incrimination.

Table 8.2 gives a detailed review of criminal laws in the former EU Member States where FGM is punishable under general criminal law.

Other legislative texts dealing (indirectly) with FGM

In all Member States, other laws exist that can be brought against FGM, such as: child protection procedures; laws that deal with doctors', other officials' and the public's reporting duty in case of (suspicion of) violence; unlawful medical practice; or texts that deal with the 'duty to help a person in danger'. Child protection procedures and laws with regard to professional secrecy are the two most important legislative texts that are indirectly tackling the practice of FGM. Table 8.3 gives an overview of existing child protection law provisions in Belgium, France, Spain, Sweden and the UK, in the case of child abuse. In these countries, there are no specific child protection provisions with regard to FGM, although in the UK, France, Sweden and Spain, guidelines for professionals have been developed with regard to protecting a child from FGM.

Social workers and health professionals can have an important role in reporting cases of suspicion of FGM being carried out, or of a girl at risk. However, in this respect it is important to know what the law says with regard to professional secrecy, i.e. if they have the duty or the right to report. Table 8.4 gives an overview of professional secrecy provisions in Belgium, France, Spain, Sweden and the UK. It indicates that professionals have a duty to report child abuse, either to social authorities (Sweden, France and the UK) or to judicial authorities (France, Spain). In Belgium, professionals do not have a duty but a right to report.

Difficulties in implementing laws[1]

Research on legal provisions in the EU showed that criminal law provisions are no guarantee for court cases, and that specific legislations are not more successful in punishing FGM than criminal law provisions. The research concluded that the implementation of laws on FGM meets two main barriers: the reporting of cases of suspicion of performed FGM and suspicion of a future performance of FGM, and

Table 8.2 General criminal law provisions applicable to FGM in former EU Member States[1]

Country	Criminal law provision	Aggravating circumstance increasing penalty	Extraterritoriality	Criminal prosecutions
Finland	Chapter 21, sections 5&6 Penal Code: assault or serious assault	Loss of essential body parts/Offence endangers life of the victim/Offence causes death	No	No
France	Article 222–9/10 of the Penal Code: mutilation	Offence against minor/Offence performed by parent, person having custody (prosecuted as accomplices)	Yes, if the victim is a French national	Yes
Germany	Sections 224 and 226 of the Penal Code: serious and grave bodily harm	Loss of essential parts of the body/Permanent and incurable corporal lesions	Yes, if the victim is a German national and exigency of double incrimination or offender is German and he/she has not been extradited to the country where the crime is committed	No
Greece	Articles 308–315 of the Penal Code: bodily injury	Offence against minor/Offence performed by parent/person having custody/Loss of essential parts of the body/Permanent and incurable corporal lesions/offence endangers life/Offence causes death	No	No
Ireland	Criminal Justice Act 2000: bodily injury	Offence against minor/Loss of essential body parts/Permanent loss of working capacity/Offence endangers life/Offence causes death	No	No

Italy	Article 583 of the Penal Code: bodily injury or serious bodily injury	Offence performed by parent, person having custody/Loss of essential parts of the body/Permanent and incurable corporal lesions	Yes, if the offender is found on the territory and if a claim is made by the victim	Yes
Luxembourg	Article 392 of the Penal Code: voluntary corporal lesion	Offence against minor/Offence performed by parent, person having custody/Loss of essential body parts/Permanent and incurable corporal lesions/Permanent loss of working capacity/Offence causes death, disease, serious mutilation/Offence carried out with premeditation	No	No
Portugal	Articles 143–149 of the Penal Code: bodily injury or serious bodily injury	Offence against minor/Offence performed by parent, person having custody/Loss of essential body parts/Permanent and incurable corporal lesions/Permanent loss of working capacity/Offence endangers life/Offence causes death	No	No
The Netherlands	Articles 300–304 of the Penal Code: bodily injury or serious bodily injury	Offence performed by parent, person having custody/Serious corporal lesions/Offence causes death	Yes. Exigency of double incrimination *and* on the condition that the offender is a national or liability for preparatory acts in the Netherlands concerning a FGM operation	No

Table 8.3 Child protection measures in Belgium, France, Spain, Sweden and the United Kingdom[1]

	Belgium	France	Spain	Sweden	United Kingdom
Child protection provision(s)	Child protection law (1965)	Article 375 of the Civil Code	Civil Code Articles 9.6, 92, 93, 156, 216.2, 217/ Parliamentary Law of Judiciary Power: Articles 22.3 and 5/National child protection laws: organic law 21/1987, 11 November and organic law 1/1996, 15 January/Autonomous Communities have their own child protection laws	Social Services Act/ Care of Young Persons Act (1990)/Act regarding Special Representative for a Child (1999)	Children Act 1989
FGM is specifically mentioned	No	No	No	No	No
A specific FGM child protection guideline is provided	No	Yes, Regional guideline applicable in Paris Information brochures disseminated nationally	Yes: Girona Protocol (only applicable in Catalonia); Interdisciplinary commission on FGM was constituted on 14/11/2003 to discuss and approve the 'Aragon Protocol'	Yes, elaborated by the Swedish Board of Health and Welfare (2002)	Yes, FGM is mentioned in the chapter entitled 'child protection in specific circumstances' elaborated by the Department of Health (1999)

Voluntary child protection measures	Hearing with the family/Informing, counselling and warning	Hearing with the family/Informing, counselling and warning	Hearing with the family/ Informing, counselling and warning	Hearing with the family/Informing, counselling and warning	Meeting with the family/Informing, counselling and warning
Compulsory child protection measures	Certain acts are subject to court permission, e.g. travel permission/ Removing child from family/ Suspending parental authority	Certain acts are subject to court permission, e.g. travel permission/Removing child from family/ Suspending parental authority	Certain acts are subject to court permission, e.g. travel permission/ Periodic medical (genital) examination of a child/ Removing child from family/Suspending parental authority	Medical (genital) examination of a child/ Removing child from family/Suspending parental authority	Certain acts are subject to court permission, e.g. travel permission/ Removing child from family/Suspending parental authority
Child protection interventions	No	Yes	Yes	Yes	Yes

Table 8.4 Professional secrecy provisions in Belgium, France, Spain, Sweden and the United Kingdom[1]

	Belgium	France	Spain	Sweden	United Kingdom
Professional secrecy provision(s)	Article 458 and 458bis of the Penal Code	Article 226-13 and 226-14 of the Penal Code Article 434-3 of the Penal Code	Article 263 of the Criminal Procedure Law	Secrecy Act (1980)	Document *Working Together to Safeguard Children* Professional guidelines
FGM is specifically mentioned	Yes	No	No	No Specific guidelines elaborated by the Swedish Board of Health and Welfare (2002)	Yes
Which professionals are envisaged?	Health professionals Other professionals bound to secrecy such as education staff and social workers	Health professionals	Lawyers; priests	Health professionals/ social authorities	Health professionals Social workers Police Education staff
Conditions for disclosing information	Article 458bis: crime of FGM is committed against minor *and* the victim is in danger *and* he/she cannot ensure the integrity of the minor	When the law imposes or authorises disclosure, e.g. in case of deprivation or abuse, including sexual harm or assault committed against a minor or any person unable to protect herself	Not specified	In case of any crime which may lead to a minimum of two years' imprisonment If the purpose is to prevent a crime	When there is a need to protect the child's welfare and safety
Duty or right to report	Right to report to prosecution authorities	Duty to report to administrative or judicial authorities	Health professionals and teachers have a duty to report to police or judicial authorities/ Citizens have an obligation to denounce to prosecutor, competent court instruction judge or police	Duty to report any suspicion of child abuse to the social authorities/ Social authorities may report a crime involving a child to the police	Duty to report to social services

the finding of sufficient evidence to bring a case to court (only in France, more than 30 cases have reached the courtroom).

The implementation of laws is further exacerbated by the fact that in some countries those health professionals, authorities and police officers who need to be alert to the problem of FGM have a lack of knowledge about the practice in general and about the legal provisions and procedures to follow in particular. Furthermore, all these actors have their own attitudes towards migrant populations and towards the practice of FGM. In the UK, for example, fieldwork showed that several professionals are paralysed into inaction because of fear being labelled 'racist'.[18]

Given the difficulties of implementing criminal laws with regard to FGM, the study argues that more attention needs to be paid to child protection measures in order to prevent girls from FGM. A particular problem in the area of child protection that needs further investigation is that of the girls that do not return from holidays (parents do not want to risk the discovery of FGM upon their return to the host country), as noted in Sweden,[17] France[24] and the UK.[18]

Developing legislation to punish a crime is one thing; the implementation of such legislation is another. The example of FGM, as examined in this research, showed that the implementation of FGM legislation is a complex issue and not an obvious or automatic process. Several actors are active at various levels (such as medical doctors, child protection officers, social workers, police officers, prosecutors, etc.), and various determinants influence the process of implementation (for example knowledge about FGM, attitudes about FGM and/or the practising communities, (lack of) consultation between the actors, etc.). Therefore, the implementation of legislation requires sufficient time, resources and (political) will in order to be successful.

Education and prevention in Europe

NGOs working towards the eradication of FGM in Europe emerged from the early eighties, such as Terre Des Femmes in Germany (founded in 1981) or the 'Groupement pour l'Abolition des Mutilations Sexuelles' in France (founded in 1982). NGOs and community-based organisations have either focused their work solely on FGM or adopted a holistic approach by incorporating the issue in their work on women's issues, health issues, or migrant/refugee issues.[22]

For example, in Sweden, Denmark, Germany, the United Kingdom, Italy and the Netherlands, a wide range of actors work at different levels of society to prevent FGM: at healthcare level, within the police, the media, at community level, schools, etc. The activities of the NGOs are devoted to prevention work, lobbying and advocacy. They provide information, education and communication activities towards the African communities and towards the Western audience. These include the production of training programs for professionals, developing educational material and developing awareness-raising campaigns aimed at different target groups. Some NGOs and community-based organisations also conduct research and give support to organisations in Africa, such as AIDOS in Italy or FORWARD in the UK.

Following two workshops organised by the International Centre for Reproductive Health in 2000, in collaboration with the Immigration Services of the City of Göteborg in Sweden, fieldworkers from 11 European countries exchanged experiences and information with regard to their approach of the prevention of FGM in their European countries of residence.

Topics that were discussed included: use of terminology during prevention work; communication with the different target groups; communication with the media; collaboration with African organisations and collaboration at national and European level; the use of educational material; training of fieldworkers; involving religious leaders; and working towards behaviour change.

Some of the conclusions of this workshop that need further attention concerned the lack of needs assessments before activities of NGOs are initiated; failing communication with the media; the lack of co-operation at national and European level; the lack of evaluations of the educational material that is used in Europe and the need to collaborate with religious leaders, youth and men.[22]

In some European countries national co-ordinating and/or advisory bodies have been established, for example in the Netherlands, where stakeholders meet regularly at national level. At European level, however, there is no common policy or co-ordinated approach with regard to the healthcare, legislations or prevention work.

In March 2002, the European Network for the Prevention and Eradication of Harmful Traditional Practices Affecting the Health of Women and Children, in Particular Female Genital Mutilation (EuroNet FGM) was founded. It joins NGOs, researchers, health professionals and activists from all over Europe.

Healthcare services in Europe[25]

Research from 1998[10] and 2000[26] showed that in Europe three main health interventions are put in place dealing with health issues related to FGM:

1 technical guidelines for the clinical management of women with FGM
2 codes of conduct for health professionals and
3 specialised health services that provide medical care, psychological care and counselling.[26]

Technical guidelines[26]

Hospitals and/or Ministries of Health in some European countries have developed technical guidelines for the clinical management of women with FGM. These guidelines deal mainly with health complications of FGM and with technical procedures to follow in case of de-infibulation, and care at the time of delivery, antenatal and post-partum care. The technical advice published in Belgium for example, for dealing with delivery procedures for infibulated women, has been published in French and Dutch and is available from the Federal Ministry of Public Health.[27]

Codes of conduct for health professionals[26]

Codes of conduct are mainly developed by professionals' organisations, such as the Dutch Society of Gynaecology and Obstetrics, who developed a position paper on female genital mutilation, as well as the British Medical Association and the Royal College of Midwives of England. These codes go beyond giving advice on the clinical management of women with FGM, as they also outline the provision of ethnically sensitive care, and give insights in the ethical and legal issues with regard to FGM and the health services.

Specialised health services[26]

In the UK, specialist midwives, often members of the affected African communities themselves, are working in African Well Woman Clinics (AWWC) that have been established in the past decade. Examples include the AWWC at Northwick Park Hospital in Middlesex established in 1993, and the AWWC at Guy's and St Thomas' in London (1995).[28,29] These services provide appropriate medical care, support, information, advice and counselling to women and their partners. They also offer de-infibulation, where appropriate, to both pregnant and non-pregnant women, and training for healthcare professionals.[26]

Specialised health services for women who have undergone FGM, however, are more the exception than the rule in Europe and guidelines and codes of conduct are not provided for in all health services. A study in Sweden,[30] for example, mentions that midwives feel a lack of supportive guidelines with regard to requests for re-infibulation.

Most general health services in Europe are unfamiliar with the consequences of FGM. This can result in inadequate care (for example, unnecessary Caesarean sections in case of infibulation) and discourages women from seeking appropriate care for their FGM-related problems. Personal emotions and feelings, such as feelings of powerlessness (as some FGM procedures are irreversible) or anger (cutting genitals is alien to Western practice), can also hamper the provision of adequate care.[26,31] The lack of knowledge about the needs and expectations of the affected communities about healthcare is also apparent, for example, in the Netherlands, where a small study revealed that obstetric care is insufficiently focused on the expectations and needs of Somali women.[26,32]

In order to provide appropriate and sensitive healthcare for women with genital mutilation, the need and health-seeking behaviour of affected communities needs to be assessed. Furthermore, healthcare professionals' training needs need to be assessed and should take into account various levels: clinical care, prevention of FGM, counselling, communication and attitudes, and ethical issues.

Guidelines on counselling services, on referrals of girls at risk or women with genital mutilation, on successful communication, on clinical care and on ethical questions such as re-infibulation and medicalisation need to be developed. And last but not least, the operational coherence between health and other agencies that are confronted with FGM should be improved by multisectoral collaboration, in order to provide adequate holistic care for women with FGM.

Research activities in Europe

The amount of research on FGM in Europe, either on clinical aspects or on social and behavioural aspects of FGM in relation to a European setting, is scarce. Such research is, however, paramount for any EU Member State's FGM policy initiatives, as such initiatives need to be based on rigorous evidence-based research if they are to be effective.[12]

At a workshop held at the International Centre for Reproductive Health (June 2000), priority research areas have been determined that focus specifically on the European setting,[12,33] some of which are included below:

Prevalence in Europe

As stated earlier in the chapter, evidence on the magnitude of the problem of FGM should be collected to show that FGM is important enough to justify taking action.

An inventory of existing interventions and their impact analysis

Interventions developed at legislative, community and health and social sector level need to be inventoried across Europe, and an evaluation of their activities undertaken to determine their relative effectiveness.[11]

Research on behavioural changes related to a migration context

More research needs to be done on those who have abandoned the practice while living in exile, in order to determine the factors of this behaviour change process and to develop more effective interventions.[12]

Conclusions

Many initiatives have been taken at various levels to tackle FGM across Europe, but some issues remain. First of all, the magnitude of the problem of FGM in Europe needs to be assessed in order to measure any progress made and to give any initiative that deals with FGM a basis in evidence.

In order for legal provisions that deal with FGM to become effective, the implementation of these laws needs more attention, especially in finding solutions to identify cases and in supplying suspected cases with sufficient evidence to bring a case to court. Furthermore, more attention needs to be paid to child protection measures in order to prevent girls from undergoing FGM.

With regard to education and prevention initiatives in Europe, issues that need further attention include co-operation at national and European level, evaluation of educational material and collaboration with specific target groups such as religious leaders, youth and men.

The need for evidence-based research and needs assessments before actions are taking place is paramount if actions are to be effective. Research in Europe should also focus on performing evaluations of existing interventions to determine their effectiveness. Assessing determinants of behaviour changes could also support the development of more effective interventions.

Health services in Europe need to assess the training needs of their professionals, develop appropriate guidelines and discuss ethical issues. The healthcare needs of the affected communities need to be assessed in order to develop culturally sensitive healthcare.

And last but not least, there is a need for a better coherence between all agencies working towards the abandonment of FGM. The European Resolution on FGM made some useful suggestions for developing a European policy with regard to FGM and it has the potential to guide the design and implementation of a common approach to deal with FGM in Europe. The European Network for the Prevention of FGM, although being relatively embryonic and lacking an adequate funding base, has the potential to put into practice the suggestions made by the Resolution and to become the consultative agency at the European level on FGM.[34]

References

1   Leye E, Deblonde J and Temmerman M (2004) *A comparative analysis of the different legal approaches in the 15 EU Member States, and the respective judicial outcomes in Belgium, France, Spain, Sweden and the United Kingdom.* The Consultory, Lokeren; ICRH Publications No 8.

2   Izett S and Toubia N (1999) *Learning about Social Change: a research and evaluation guidebook using female circumcision as a case study.* Rainbo, New York.

3   Délégation Régionale aux Droits des Femmes (1998) *Dossier de présentation du dépliant: Agir face aux mutilations sexuelles féminines relatif à la prévention.* Préfecture d'Ile-de-France, Paris.

4   Equilibres et Populations (2003) La prévention ne doit pas faire oublier la réparation. *Equilibres et Populations.* Supp. au No. 88. Décembre 2003–Janvier 2004. p. 4.

5   Utz B (2000) German guidelines for health care professionals. In: E Leye and A Githaiga (eds) *Workshop report 'Female genital mutilation in Europe: developing frameworks for the health care sector'.* International Centre for Reproductive Health, Ghent.

6   Grassivaro Gallo P, Livio M and Viviani F (1995) Survey on Italian obstetricians and gynaecologists: FGM in African immigrants. In: P Grassivaro Gallo and F Viviani (eds) *FGM: a public health issue also in Italy.* Unipress, Padua.

7   Grassivaro Gallo P, Araldi L and Viviani F (2001) Genital mutilation among female adolescents resident in Italy. *The Mankin Quarterly XLII.* **2**: 155–68.

8   Jäger F, Schulze S and Hohlfeld P (2002). Female genital mutilation in Switzerland: a survey among gynaecologists. *Swiss Medical Weekly.* **132**: 259–64.

9   Read D (1998) *Out of sight, out of mind?* Forward, London.

10 Leye E, de Bruyn M and Meuwese S (2003) *Proceedings of the expert meeting on female genital mutilation.* Ghent, Belgium, 5–7 November 1998. The Consultory, Lokeren; ICRH Publications No 2.

11 Leye E (2001) The struggle against female genital mutilation/female circumcision: the European experience. In: GC Denniston, F Mansfield Hodges and MF Milos (eds) *Understanding circumcision: a multidisciplinary approach to a multi-dimensional problem.* Kluwer Academic/Plenum Publishers, New York.

12 Powell RA, Leye E and Jayakody A *et al.* (2004) Female genital mutilation, asylum seekers and refugees: the need for an integrated European Union agenda. *Health Policy.* **70**: 151–62.

13 World Health Organization (2001) *Female genital mutilation: a teacher's guide.* World Health Organization, Geneva.

14 Abi Ahmed L, Ndiaye Diye and Cubattoli C *et al.* (no date) *Progetto 'Iman'. Sintesi del rapporto di ricerca sulle MGF.* Nosotras, Firenze.

15 Leye E and Deblonde J (2004) *Belgian legislation regarding female genital mutilation and the implementation of the law in Belgium.* ICRH Publications No 9, The Consultory, Lokeren.

16 De Lucas J, Añón Roig MJ, Bedoya MH *et al* (2004) *Evaluating the impact of existing legislation in Europe with regard to FGM. Spanish national report.* Centre of Studies on Citizenship, Migration and Minorities, University of Valencia, Valencia.

17 Johnsdotter S (2003) *FGM in Sweden. Swedish legislation regarding 'female genital mutilation' and implementation of the law.* Lund University, Lund.

18 Kwateng-Kluvitse A (2004) *UK's legislation regarding female genital mutilation and the implementation of the law in the UK.* Forward, London.
19 Rahman A and Toubia N (eds) (2000) *Female genital mutilation: a guide to laws and policies worldwide.* Zed Books/CRLP & Rainbow, New York.
20 Smith J (1995) *Visions and discussions on genital mutilation of girls. An international survey.* Defence for Children International, Amsterdam.
21 Leye E, Deblonde J and Temmerman M (2004) Vrouwenbesnijdenis in Europa. Enkele knelpunten bij de aanpak van de gezondheidszorg, wetgeving en preventiewerk. *Ethiek en Maatschappij.* **7**(4): 40–54.
22 Leye E (2000) *Report of the Gothenburg workshops 'Exchanging experiences and information at community level'.* Gothenburg April and September 2000. International Centre for Reproductive Health, Ghent.
23 Leye E, Deblonde J and Temmerman M (2004) *A comparative analysis of the different legal approaches in the 15 EU Member States, and the respective judicial outcomes in Belgium, France, Spain, Sweden and the United Kingdom.* The Consultory, Lokeren; ICRH Publications No 8.
24 Weil-Curiel L (2004) *French legislation regarding FGM and the implementation of the law in France.* CAMS, Paris.
25 Leye E, Powell RA, Nienhuis G *et al.* (2005) Health care in Europe for women with genital mutilation. Accepted for publication to *Health Care for Women International.*
26 Leye, E and Githaiga A (2000) *Workshop Report: 'Female genital mutilation in Europe: developing frameworks for the health sector'.* Ghent, 15–17 June 2000. International Centre for Reproductive Health, Ghent.
27 Richard F, Daniel D, Ostyn B *et al.* (2000) *Technisch advies voor gezondheidspersoneel in België. Vrouwelijke genitale verminking (vrouwenbesnijdenis). Handleiding bij de bevalling.* Ministry of Health, Brussels.
28 McCaffrey M, Jankowska A and Gordon H (1995) Management of female genital mutilation: the Northwick Park Hospital experience. *Br J Obstet Gynaecol.* **102**: 787–90.
29 Momoh C, Ladhani S, Lochrie DP *et al.* (2001) Female genital mutilation: analysis of the first twelve months of a Southeast London specialist clinic. *Br J Obstet Gynaecol.* **108**: 186–91.
30 Widmark C, Tishelman C and Ahlberg BM (2002) A study of Swedish midwives' encounters with infibulated African women in Sweden. *Midwifery.* **18**: 113–25.
31 Nienhuis G and Haaijer I (1995) Ignorance of female circumcision may hamper adequate care. In: Werkgroep Interculturele Verpleging (ed.) *Intercultureel Verplegen.* De Tijdstroom, Utrecht.
32 Nienhuis G (1998) Somali women tell: It's like you have to do the delivery here by yourself. *Tijdschrift voor Verloskundigen.* **23**: 160–6.
33 Leye E (2000) *Workshop report «Female genital mutilation in Europe: setting a research agenda».* Ghent, 22–23 June 2000. International Centre for Reproductive Health, Ghent.
34 Leye E, Deblonde J and Temmerman M (2004) Vrouwenbesnijdenis in Europa. Enkele knelpunten in de aanpak van de gezondheidszorg, wetgeving en preventie. *Ethiek en Maatschappij.* **7**(4): 40–54.

Chapter Nine

Attitudes towards FGM among Somali women living in the UK

Marwa Ahmed

Introduction

As identified in other chapters, female genital mutilation (FGM) or female circumcision is widely practised, mainly in Africa and the Middle East. It also occurs in the West, mainly among immigrant communities. In Somalia, 98% of women would have undergone some form of FGM, mainly the infibulation type.[1,2] *See* 10, colour plate section for a map of Africa showing Somalia to illustrate the area featured in this chapter.[3]

A raising of awareness and education about FGM is essential for women in areas with a high prevalence of FGM, and among health and social care professionals and those working in statutory and voluntary organisations everywhere. There is also a need for qualitative research into the psychosocial effects of FGM if we are to identify ways that health professionals can contribute to care provision.

One has to explore the influence of cross-cultural psychology, women's experience of FGM and their attitudes towards it. This chapter aims to reflect the views of Somali women, living in the UK, towards the practice of FGM. Autobiographical accounts of the day they underwent FGM are included. In addition, how health professionals in the UK might be able to help such women with their medical, as well as psychological needs in order to stop such a practice from continuing through future generations.

Study methodology

Seven focus groups were conducted. Each group composed of 7–9 participants between 18–70 years of age. They were recruited via word of mouth, through attending Somali community centres and verbal advertising of the project. Groups one and two were interviewed in White City in the West of London. Group three was interviewed in Bermondsey in South East of London. Groups four, five and six were interviewed in Pitsmore in Sheffield. Group seven was interviewed in Brixton in South London.

Participants were interviewed in a focus group setting, and the meetings were conducted in English, Somali or Arabic. A majority of the meetings took place in the women's homes, as they preferred a private and familiar atmosphere, interviews five and six took place in a community centre and interview seven was held in a mosque. Meetings lasted between 45 minutes and 2 hours. Participants were firstly asked a series of general questions such as their age, marital status, length of stay in the UK and place of birth.

They were then asked about their life experiences in the UK and eventually the discussions led to FGM. Each participant was asked whether they had experienced FGM. If yes, at what age and whether they knew which type. Then followed general questions designed to elicit their views about FGM and whether living in the UK has altered any of their opinions. Since men's involvement in the decision making is largely ignored in research, the women were asked about it. In the meetings, either 'female circumcision' or the Somali version of the word were used instead of FGM, as women weren't aware of the term FGM.

A data-driven approach was used. The discussions were tape recorded, transcribed immediately after the meetings and subjected to thematic analysis, using the method of Boyatzis.[4] Transcripts were shortened into outlines per transcript, which divided each transcript into four main themes and then summarised the important phrases and issues raised by participants under each theme. Themes were then recorded into a table format, again divided into two categories, depending on age and marital status. The first group was made up of 18- to 30-year-old single participants. The second group was composed of 31- to 70-year-old participants, and those who were married, divorced or widowed regardless of their age. Cross tabulation of personal information of the participants along with their opinions was also performed.

Study results

Demographics of participants

Table 9.1   The age of the participants

Age	Frequency	Percent	Valid percent
Over 30	1	1.8	1.8
N/A	3	5.4	5.4
18	8	14.3	14.3
19	2	3.6	3.6
20	3	5.4	5.4
21	2	3.6	3.6
22	4	7.1	7.1
23	1	1.8	1.8
24	1	1.8	1.8
27	5	8.9	8.9
28	3	5.4	5.4
31	2	3.6	3.6
33	2	3.6	3.6
34	1	1.8	1.8
35	3	5.4	5.4
37	1	1.8	1.8
39	1	1.8	1.8
42	1	1.8	1.8
43	1	1.8	1.8
44	1	1.8	1.8
50	3	5.4	5.4
56	1	1.8	1.8
58	1	1.8	1.8
59	1	1.8	1.8
60	3	5.4	5.4
70	1	1.8	1.8
Total	**56**	**100.0**	**100.0**

Table 9.2 Place of birth of the participants

Place of birth	Frequency	Percent
Berbera	1	1.8
Mogadishu	14	25.0
Burco	11	19.6
North Somalia	3	5.4
Kuwait	1	1.8
Doha	1	1.8
UK	1	1.8
Sheffield	1	1.8
Scotland	1	1.8
Bolton	1	1.8
Leeds	1	1.8
Yemen	1	1.8
Somalia	2	3.6
Afgoya	1	1.8
Saudi Arabia	1	1.8
Dubai	2	3.6
Hargeysa	10	17.9
N/A	3	5.4
Total	**56**	**100.0**

The recruited participants were between the ages of 18 and 70 years. The majority were born in Burco and Hargeysa in the North of Somalia and in Mogadishu in the South. The rest were born in Somalia, UK and the Middle East. N/A refers to the number of participants who didn't give any information.

Table 9.3 Marital status of the participants

Marital status	Frequency	Percent
Single	27	48.2
Married	15	26.8
Divorced	3	5.4
Widow	5	8.9
N/A	5	8.9
Engaged	1	1.8
Total	**56**	**100.0**

The majority of these participants were single or married. They lived in different areas in the UK, as shown, but the majority lived in Pitsmore in Sheffield and in White City in the West of London.

Table 9.4   Participants' length of stay in the UK

Length of stay in UK (Years)	Frequency	Percent
0.3	2	3.6
0.5	1	1.8
0.7	1	1.8
1.0	3	5.4
1.8	1	1.8
2.0	3	5.4
3.0	4	7.1
4.0	4	7.1
6.0	1	1.8
7.0	1	1.8
7.5	1	1.8
8.0	4	7.1
9.0	1	1.8
10.0	3	5.4
11.0	3	5.4
12.0	4	7.1
14.0	7	12.5
15.0	1	1.8
17.0	1	1.8
Born in UK	5	8.9
N/A	4	7.1
38.0	1	1.8
Total	**56**	**100.0**

There was a variation in the length of stay in the UK among the recruited participants. This varied from four months (0.3 years) to 38 years, and some of the participants were born in the UK in places such as Sheffield and Bolton.

FGM characteristics of participants

Table 9.5   The type of FGM the women underwent

Type of FGM	Frequency	Percent
Not FGM	3	5.4
Type 1 (SUNNA)	14	25.0
Type 3 (INFIBULATION)	35	62.5
N/A	3	5.4
Type 2	1	1.8
Total	**56**	**100.0**

62.5% of participants have undergone Type 3 infibulation compared to 25% who have undergone clitoridectomy/Sunna, and only 1.8% have undergone Type 2, which is an extension of Type 1.

Table 9.6 The type of FGM the women underwent according to their age

Statistics: count		Type of FGM				
Age	Not FGM	Type 1 (Sunna)	Type 3 (Infibulation)	N/A	Type 2	Total
Over 30	0	0	1	0	0	1
N/A	0	0	3	0	0	3
18	2	3	2	0	1	8
19	1	1	0	0	0	2
20	0	3	0	0	0	3
21	0	1	1	0	0	2
22	0	2	2	0	0	4
23	0	0	1	0	0	1
24	0	1	0	0	0	1
27	0	1	1	3	0	5
28	0	0	3	0	0	3
31	0	0	2	0	0	2
33	0	0	2	0	0	2
34	0	0	1	0	0	1
35	0	0	3	0	0	3
37	0	0	1	0	0	1
39	0	0	1	0	0	1
42	0	0	1	0	0	1
43	0	0	1	0	0	1
44	0	0	1	0	0	1
50	0	1	2	0	0	3
56	0	0	1	0	0	1
58	0	1	0	0	0	1
59	0	0	1	0	0	1
60	0	0	3	0	0	3
70	0	0	1	0	0	1
Total	**3**	**14**	**35**	**3**	**1**	**56**

Of the 62.5% who have undergone Type 3, the majority were over the age of 30 (n = 22) compared to those under 30 (n = 10). In terms of Type 1, the majority who have undergone this procedure were under the age of 30 (n = 12), and only two were over the age of 30 (n = 2). Only one participant aged 18 had undergone Type 2. There were three participants who had not undergone FGM, since they had moved to Holland from Somalia at a young age.

Table 9.7   The influence of place of birth on the type of FGM

Count		Type of FGM				
Place of birth	Not FGM	Type 1 (Sunna)	Type 3 (Infibulation)	N/A	Type 2	Total
Berbera	0	0	1	0	0	1
Mogadishu	0	4	9	1	0	14
Burco	0	0	11	0	0	11
North Somalia	0	0	3	0	0	3
Kuwait	0	1	0	0	0	1
Doha	0	0	1	0	0	1
UK	0	1	0	0	0	1
Sheffield	0	1	0	0	0	1
Scotland	0	1	0	0	0	1
Bolton	0	1	0	0	0	1
Leeds	0	1	0	0	0	1
Yemen	0	0	1	0	0	1
Somalia	0	0	1	0	1	2
Afgoya	0	0	1	0	0	1
Saudi Arabia	0	0	0	1	0	1
Dubai	1	1	0	0	0	2
Hargeysa	2	1	6	1	0	10
N/A	0	2	1	0	0	3
Total	**3**	**14**	**35**	**3**	**1**	**56**

Those who have had Type 3 were born mainly in Mogadishu in the South of Somalia, Burco and Hargeysa in the North. Those who have undergone Type 1 were mainly born outside Somalia either in the Middle East or in the UK (n = 7), or they were born in Mogadishu (n = 4). Those who were not FGM were born in Hargeysa or Dubai; however, they emigrated from Somalia to Holland at a very young age.

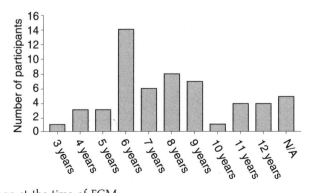

Figure 9.1   Age at the time of FGM

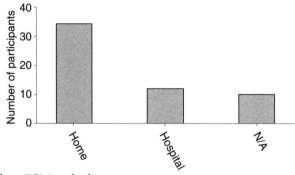

Figure 9.2 Where FGM took place

The participants had undergone FGM between the age of six and nine, with the majority undergoing FGM at the age of six (n = 14). The procedure of FGM had taken place at home in 60.7% (34) of the participants, compared to 21.4% in hospital (n = 12)

Table 9.8 The influence of place of birth on where FGM took place

Statistics: count	Where FGM took place			
Place of birth	Home	Hospital	N/A	Total
Berbera	1	0	0	1
Mogadishu	5	6	3	14
Burco	8	1	2	11
North Somalia	2	1	0	3
Kuwait	1	0	0	1
Doha	1	0	0	1
UK	1	0	0	1
Sheffield	0	0	1	1
Scotland	1	0	0	1
Bolton	0	1	0	1
Leeds	1	0	0	1
Yemen	1	0	0	1
Somalia	2	0	0	2
Afgoya	1	0	0	1
Saudi Arabia	1	0	0	1
Dubai	0	1	1	2
Hargeysa	7	1	2	10
N/A	1	1	1	3
Total	**34**	**12**	**10**	**56**

Most of the participants seemed to have undergone FGM at home, whether they were born in Somalia, the Middle East or in the UK. In areas in the North of Somalia, such as Hargeysa, Berbera and Burco, women seemed to have been FGM at home compared to the South in Mogadishu, where almost an equal number of women got FGM in hospital and at home. All those who were born in the UK except one underwent FGM at home, due to the practice being illegal in the UK; some were taken on holiday to the Middle East to undergo FGM.

Factors influencing participants' opinions

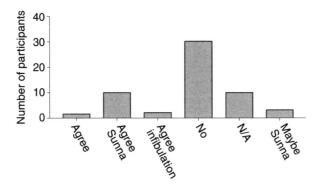

Figure 9.3   The opinion of the women regarding FGM

53.6% of participants (n = 30) were against the practice of any form of FGM compared to 17.9% who supported clitoridectomy/Sunna (n = 10) and only 3.6% who supported Type 3 infibulation (n = 2). However, 5.4% were considering Type 1 Sunna (n = 3).

Table 9.9 The influence of age on the opinion

Count				Opinion			
Age	Agree	Agree (Sunna)	Agree (Infibulation)	No	N/A	Maybe (Sunna)	Total
Over 30	0	0	0	1	0	0	1
N/A	0	1	0	1	1	0	3
18	0	0	0	5	1	2	8
19	0	0	0	2	0	0	2
20	0	0	0	2	1	0	3
21	0	1	0	0	1	0	2
22	0	1	0	2	0	1	4
23	0	0	0	1	0	0	1
24	0	1	0	0	0	0	1
27	0	0	0	2	3	0	5
28	0	3	0	0	0	0	3
31	0	0	0	0	2	0	2
33	0	2	0	0	0	0	2
34	0	0	0	0	1	0	1
35	0	0	0	3	0	0	3
37	0	0	0	1	0	0	1
39	0	0	0	1	0	0	1
42	0	0	0	1	0	0	1
43	0	0	0	1	0	0	1
44	0	0	1	0	0	0	1
50	0	1	0	2	0	0	3
56	0	0	0	1	0	0	1
58	0	0	0	1	0	0	1
59	0	0	1	0	0	0	1
60	1	0	0	2	0	0	3
70	0	0	0	1	0	0	1
Total	**1**	**10**	**2**	**30**	**10**	**3**	**56**

53.6% (n = 30) do not support FGM. There seems to be no influence of age on this opinion, since 14 participants under 30 were against this practice compared to 15 over 30. However, for those who supported FGM (n = 10), six under the age of 30 supported Type 1, and two over the age of 30 supported Type 3. Finally, three participants under the age of 30 did not have a definite opinion but they were considering support for Type 1.

Table 9.10 The influence of place of birth on the opinion

Count			Opinion				
Place of birth	Agree	Agree (Sunna)	Agree (Infibulation)	No	N/A	Maybe (Sunna)	Total
Berbera, Somalia	0	0	0	1	0	0	1
Mogadishu, Somalia	0	6	1	5	1	1	14
Burco, Somalia	1	0	1	6	2	1	11
North Somalia	0	2	0	1	0	0	3
Kuwait	0	0	0	1	0	0	1
Doha, Qatar	0	0	0	1	0	0	1
UK	0	0	0	0	0	1	1
Sheffield, UK	0	0	0	1	0	0	1
Scotland, UK	0	0	0	1	0	0	1
Bolton, UK	0	0	0	1	0	0	1
Leeds, UK	0	0	0	1	0	0	1
Yemen	0	0	0	1	0	0	1
Somalia	0	0	0	1	1	0	2
Afgoya, Somalia	0	0	0	1	0	0	1
Saudi Arabia	0	0	0	0	1	0	1
Dubai, UAE	0	0	0	1	1	0	2
Hargeysa, Somalia	0	1	0	6	3	0	10
N/A	0	1	0	1	1	0	3
Total	**1**	**10**	**2**	**30**	**10**	**3**	**56**

In terms of those who opposed FGM, they were mainly born in Mogadishu in the South, or in the North such as Burco and Hargeysa. All those who were born in the UK and the Middle East opposed it too, except for a British-born participant who considered support for Type 1 Sunna. Those who supported Type 1 were born in Mogadishu and Hargeysa, and those who supported Type 3 were born in Burco and again in Mogadishu.

Table 9.11 The influence of the length of stay in the UK on the opinion

Count	Opinion						
Length of stay in the UK	*Agree*	*Agree (Sunna)*	*Agree (Infibulation)*	*No*	*N/A*	*Maybe (Sunna)*	*Total*
0.3	0	2	0	0	0	0	2
0.5	0	0	0	1	0	0	1
0.7	0	0	0	0	1	0	1
1.0	0	0	0	3	0	0	3
1.8	0	0	0	1	0	0	1
2.0	0	1	0	0	2	0	3
3.0	0	0	0	3	1	0	4
4.0	0	1	0	2	1	0	4
6.0	0	1	0	0	0	0	1
7.0	0	0	0	1	0	0	1
7.5	0	0	0	1	0	0	1
8.0	0	0	1	2	0	1	4
9.0	0	0	0	0	0	1	1
10.0	0	2	0	1	0	0	3
11.0	0	0	0	3	0	0	3
12.0	0	0	0	3	1	0	4
14.0	1	0	1	3	2	0	7
15.0	0	0	0	0	1	0	1
17.0	0	0	0	0	1	0	1
Born in UK	0	0	0	4	0	1	5
N/A	0	3	0	1	0	0	4
38.0	0	0	0	1	0	0	1
Total	**1**	**10**	**2**	**30**	**10**	**3**	**56**

The length of stay in the UK did not influence the opposition and support for the practice of FGM. Whether the participant was here for six months (0.5 years), 10 years or 38 years, they were still opposed to it. The same phenomenon was observed in those who agreed or were considering Type 1 clitoridectomy/Sunna.

Table 9.12   The influence of marital status on the opinion

Count				Opinion			
Marital status	Agree	Agree (Sunna)	Agree (Infibulation)	No	N/A	Maybe (Sunna)	Total
Single	0	5	0	15	4	3	27
Married	0	2	1	8	4	0	15
Divorced	0	2	0	1	0	0	3
N/A	0	1	0	3	1	0	5
Widow	1	0	1	3	0	0	5
Engaged	0	0	0	0	1	0	1
Total	**1**	**10**	**2**	**30**	**10**	**3**	**56**

The marital status of the participants did not influence their opinion. In terms of whether they disagreed with FGM, 15 single women were opposed to it compared to 12 who were married, divorced or widowed. In terms of those who supported any form of FGM, 8 single participants compared to 7 married, divorced or widowed supported either Sunna or infibulation or considered supporting the Sunna type.

Table 9.13   The influence of the age at which FGM took place on the opinion

Statistics: Count				Opinion			
Age at time of FGM	Agree	Agree (Sunna)	Agree (Infibulation)	No	N/A	Maybe (Sunna)	Total
3 years	0	0	0	1	0	0	1
4 years	0	1	0	0	1	1	3
5 years	0	0	0	2	1	0	3
6 years	0	6	0	5	2	1	14
7 years	0	1	0	3	1	1	6
8 years	0	1	1	4	2	0	8
9 years	0	1	0	4	2	0	7
10 years	0	0	0	1	0	0	1
11 years	0	0	0	4	0	0	4
12 years	1	0	1	2	0	0	4
N/A	0	0	0	4	1	0	5
Total	**1**	**10**	**2**	**30**	**10**	**3**	**56**

The age at which FGM took place did not influence the number of participants opposing this practice. However, those who mainly supported this practice were the ones who have undergone FGM at the modal age of 6–9 years.

Table 9.14 The comparison of the influence of FGM type and where FGM took place on the opinion

Opinion			Home	Hospital	N/A	Total
			\[FGM place\]			
Agree	FGM	Type 3 (Infibulation)	1			1
	Total		1			1
Agree Sunna	FGM	Type 1 (Sunna)	2	1	0	3
		Type 3 (Infibulation)	3	2	2	7
	Total		5	3	2	10
Agree Infibulation	FGM	Type 3 (Infibulation)	2			2
	Total		2			2
No	FGM	Type Not FGM	0	0	3	3
		Type 1 (Sunna)	3	4	1	8
		Type 3 (Infibulation)	15	3	1	19
	Total		18	7	5	30
N/A	FGM	Type 1 (Sunna)	1	1	0	2
		Type 3 (Infibulation)	1	1	2	4
		N/A	2	0	1	3
		Type 2	1	0	0	1
	Total		5	2	3	10
Maybe Sunna	FGM	Type 1 (Sunna)	1			1
		Type 3 (Infibulation)	2			2
	Total		3			3

Those who opposed the practice of FGM were the ones who have undergone Type 3 infibulation at home (n = 15).

Table 9.15 The influence of location of residence on the opinion

Count					
	\[Location\]				
Opinion	White City, West London	Bermondsey, SE London	Brixton, SE London	Pitsmore, Sheffield	Total
Agree	0	1	0	0	1
Agree Sunna	7	0	2	1	10
Agree Infibulation	0	1	1	0	2
No	5	5	5	15	30
N/A	1	1	0	8	10
Maybe Sunna	2	0	0	1	3
Total	**15**	**8**	**8**	**25**	**56**

Residents of White City in West London were the only ones that strongly supported Type 1 Sunna compared to the other areas of interview, which all strongly opposed FGM. This was due to lack of awareness or any campaign against the practice of FGM.

Four main themes emerging from discussions

Theme 1: Life experiences in the UK

This discussed general issues such as language problems, housing and specific issues such as racism and culture clash. This examined their experiences and what they faced, which was influenced by their age.

'... Only problem with English language.'
'Confused, you don't know a lot about your country. You are Somali, but you don't feel like you are Somali sometimes.'

Theme 2: Participants and other women's FGM experience

This described their experiences before FGM took place, at the time of FGM, and any complications faced following it. Part of this discussed their wedding night, pregnancy and labour, which couldn't be applied to the single 18–30 age group, since sex outside marriage is forbidden in Islam and Somali culture.

'... Sharpening the knife, then in one go she cut everything off.'
'I didn't feel any pain, they gave me an injection and I was sedated.'
'... Really, I don't want to remember that, it is hurting me.'

Theme 3: Reasons for FGM

This included their reasons for FGM, through their prior knowledge or what they were told at that time.

'Because girls are horny.'
'... People will shame us and point at us.'
'... Is a must in our religion.'

Theme 4: Men's involvement in the practice of FGM

The role of men, as told by the participants, was discussed in terms of decision making at the time FGM was carried out and their attitudes towards women who are or are not FGM.

'... He was against it.'
'My dad knew about it because he went to get the lady.'

Discussions and recommendations

FGM is a widespread practice. As women and their families have migrated from FGM-practising countries to the West and presented themselves to physicians with FGM-related morbidity, the level of awareness and concerns internationally about FGM, as a cultural practice and a human rights issue, has grown over the past decade.[5]

Although the participants were born in different areas of the world aside from Somalia, they still experienced FGM. This showed that the practice of FGM was not only confined to Somalia, but took place in other areas of the world with Somali residents, including the UK. The practice of infibulation was confined to Somalia and mainly among the older generation who resided there, where clitori-dectomy was practised in the younger generations who resided outside Somalia. The age and the location at which FGM took place have not been influenced by the place of birth.

In the actual study, participants were numbered and grouped, but here some have been given a letter only.

There were four main themes.

Theme 1 explored participants' life experiences in the UK. Both groups have complained of racism and abuse, whether verbal or physical and discrimina-tion towards their religious beliefs and practices. Participant A was spat on and had her scarf removed twice; Participant B had her car broken into and her house burgled. There was a clear distinction between the overall experiences, as there was a clear difference in opinions, as related to the age group and marital status.

The single, 18–30 group (n = 24) seemed to have adapted. The majority either were born in the UK (n = 5), had been living here for more than eight years (n = 8), or had migrated to the UK from Holland, where they had resided for more than 11 years (Participants C, D, E). This group was happy here, as they were afforded education and work opportunities and they felt independent. Since they were living in surroundings very different to where they grew up, or different in culture to their parents, they faced cultural conflicts. Some felt isolated from the Somali community, as their daily life habits and ideology did not agree with the majority of the older Somali residents.

As one participant of 18 years, who has been in the UK for 12 years, expressed it:

> I feel more adapted to the British way more than the Somali way, because I grew up here.

An 18 year-old British-born participant expressed the following:

> A culture shock, because there never used to be Somalis before, because before we were free and I can walk the streets with no one bothering me but now they are all watching you and I don't like it because I am not used to it.

They dealt with these cultural differences by getting on with daily life and by trying to adapt, as much as possible, to the Western lifestyle. In addition, they got closer to the Somali community through attendance at community events and by dressing the way Somalis do, so as not to feel different. In contrast, the 30–70 group's main concerns were the lack of aid offered by social services and the government and communication and language barriers, especially when attending hospital and official appointments. This can pose a problem, as discussions of private matters with family members who may be your translator can prove difficult.

They found it much harder than the younger group to adapt to Western lifestyle and changes that followed it. According to one:

> It is not easy for us to adapt to changes with religion or tradition.

And another emphasised:

> If you work with British, they find it difficult to understand your culture or religion, what you believe. They think you have to behave like them or impress them.

All these experiences are considered to be a form of acculturation. This is defined as:

> Those phenomena, which result when groups of individuals having different cultures come into continuous first-hand contact with subsequent changes in the original culture patterns of either or both groups.[6]

This is linked with this theme, as these women have migrated from different areas of the world and settled in the UK, or they were born in the UK and had to integrate into both Somali and British cultures.

It was interesting to note that the majority of the younger participants, regardless of their place of birth, had an interest in their own culture while they interacted and accepted the Western way of life; therefore, they have chosen subconsciously the integration strategy of the acculturation process. In comparison, the older age group were more resistant to change, they came here at an older age, and with more knowledge of their culture, so when they were faced with change, they held on to their values and beliefs. So this group have chosen the separation/segregation strategy of acculturation.

Theme 2 discussed the experiences of the women before, during and after FGM, and any complications or problems they faced with their periods, pregnancy and/or labour, for example. On the preparation leading to FGM, some were told by their mothers that they were about to undergo FGM or they chose to undergo FGM. In contrast, some participants were offered no explanation, such as the British-born girls who were taken 'on holiday' to undergo FGM.

They still remembered the day FGM took place, as it was a major event in their lives. Those who underwent infibulation, especially when thorns or stitches were used to close the wound, when no pain relief was used, or when the procedure had to be repeated because the first attempt wasn't successful, seemed to remember it in explicit detail. Both groups agreed that the process of FGM was painful, either at the time of FGM or when the pain relief wore off, since it was a surgical procedure that often was practised by an unqualified woman.

In terms of clitoridectomy, participants who underwent this have either faced no problems at all, or an initial burning sensation on passing urine. Participants who underwent infibulation complained of burning sensation and problems with passing urine, severe period pain, developed kidney infection and bled following the procedure. This accumulation of urine resulted, in some cases, in bloated abdomen, and great urgency to pass urine, which the participant might not be able to do, which causes great discomfort and distress.

Specific topics were discussed with the married women to explore the effect of FGM. The infibulated women were either opened at hospital by a medical practitioner, by a woman on her wedding night, or by the husband. Those who suffered the most were women who were opened by their husbands. They either developed infection, or were not opened fully to allow comfortable sexual intercourse.

When they presented to hospital during labour, they had to be cut further to allow the baby to be delivered vaginally. In some cases this was not possible, so Caesarean section was performed. Some women were not able to have children, or suffered from fibroids and ovarian cysts, which they blamed on FGM, due to the accumulation of menstrual blood and urine, secondary to a very small introitus left after infibulation.

These complications, whether immediate or long-term, were supported by other similar remarks, which were illustrated by Cook et al.[7] and Nawal Nour,[8] and indicated by Royal College of Obstetricians and Gynaecologists.[1] Cook et al. have attributed the long-term complications women faced to the type of FGM they underwent, in particular Type 3, where a small hole was usually left, making them more susceptible to infection.

This hardship that had to be endured by these women was for various reasons, as described by **Theme 3**. Regardless of their age and place of birth, both groups agreed that the reasons that FGM was carried out, as explained to them, or as they heard, were mainly due to the procedure being part of their religious practice, culture and tradition. FGM was also a way of being accepted into the community, since everyone was carrying it out at the time, and if the parents didn't perform it on their daughter, the family would be isolated from the society and the daughter would be regarded as shameful.

If a girl was not circumcised, it was believed that she would not marry a Somali man, as men preferred them to be so. There were few opinions that were different between both groups. The older group believed that if girls were not circumcised, they would be promiscuous, bringing shame on their families. Since virginity is an important issue in the Somali culture and religious practice, FGM was seen as a solution to this problem.

In comparison, the younger group were more concerned about issues like not being labelled within the community and that FGM was seen as a transitional route to becoming a woman. Some of the older women preferred FGM, as they expressed that FGM makes the woman's genitalia look nicely presented. Finally, in Somalia, if a girl were not circumcised, she would not be able to slaughter animals, which was the main duty of the Somali women, further isolating her from society.

It was for these reasons that women accepted the act of FGM and endured the pain and the problems they faced. Some have actually chosen to be circumcised, as one 27-year-old articulated:

> I told my mum that I wanted it, because I didn't want to be the odd one out, because everyone else had it done to all the girls I knew who I used to play with, then I thought that I wanted it to be done. Then

when I had it done I told everyone that I was 'Halal', I thought that it was fantastic.

Three participants between the age of 18 and 19 years were not circumcised. They had recently immigrated to the UK from Holland, where they had spent most of their young lives. The reason they were not circumcised was due to their parents' refusal, as they were under no pressure from the community to practise this procedure, since the number of Somali residents where they lived was very small.

An area that is usually neglected in research is the men's involvement in the decision making. There were no men to interview, but through the accounts given by the participants, **Theme 4 developed, which explored the men's involvement**. For all, the father or the man who was the head of the family at that time was not present at home on the day FGM took place, or he was not involved in the decision making. Mothers always made the decision, because the girl is the mother's responsibility.

Some men agreed to their daughters being circumcised for the same reasons as given by the participants, but they were more concerned about tradition and preservation of honour of the family to ensure the girl is wed. Those who did not agree with this procedure did so due to their understanding of the health risks that followed it, or due to their religious beliefs and practices where they found no support in religion to the act of FGM.

There were a few comments by some participants that there may be a change in the attitudes of men towards FGM. According to one 50 year-old,

> Men of old days liked circumcised women, but men of today they may not like it, like the young girls who don't like it, who wouldn't do it to their daughters and don't care what the men say and it will carry on like that.

One 22 year-old said:

> Most of the guys who are my friends are totally against this kind of thing.

This was shown to be true in Sudan as well, where young men decided not to perform FGM on their daughters.[9] Regardless of their age, place of birth, marital status and length of stay in the UK, 53.6% (n = 30) were against the practice of any form of FGM. However, most participants who disagreed with FGM underwent infibulation at home. This strong opposition to FGM could be due to the complications faced following the procedure, as mentioned above. Furthermore, according to the participants, some of the reasons why women's attitudes changed were due to the extensive education women were offered, whether in the UK or Somalia, from communities and organisations who campaigned against FGM.

Now, women seek knowledge and understanding instead of blindly following traditional practices without the requirement for a rational explanation. The rising rate of formal education was shown to be a useful method in reducing the overall prevalence of FGM among Nigerian Ibo girls, as shown by Nkwo et al.[10] and discussed by Snow.[11]

The effectiveness of this campaign was obvious in all areas where interviews took place, except the residents of White City in West London, who strongly supported Type 1, which was due to the lack of awareness or any campaign against the practice of FGM and its health risks, as well as not knowing that there was no religious basis for this practice. So this further emphasises the importance of knowledge and education among women from areas with high prevalence. Similar to findings by Almroth et al.,[9] the participants' support for FGM moved from infibulation to clitoridectomy, again due to the complications faced by those with infibulation.

The participants were keen that this education be concentrated on the young generation, since some of the older ones would not change due to deeply rooted cultural practices. Part of this education is the involvement of religious leaders, which was seen as necessary, since one of the main reasons behind FGM was the belief that it is a religious obligation. Many realised, regardless of their age, that there were no religious grounds for FGM, and they urged the eradication of such a practice by continuous religious teaching for both men and women.

As the participants pointed out, FGM should not become criminalised, since it was seen as an act of protection and security by the parents for their daughters' future. Instead, the psychological and medical consequences of FGM need to be highlighted, through local campaigns and regular seminars. However, when the new law published in 2004 regarding the prohibition of the practice of FGM on any residents or UK nationals anywhere in the world was put across to the participants during the meetings, some changed their position on the practice in order not to get in trouble with the law.

So the introduction of legal papers can act as a deterrent. However, some women warned that this may drive others who still support this practice to resort to illegitimate methods regardless, to fulfil their beliefs. Therefore, before the Government introduces legal documents, they should explain thoroughly the reasons behind their publication and what they are trying to achieve.

Many participants were not happy with the services offered and provided by health professionals during their consultations or labour. One participant recalled:

> I went to hospital, I got opened, the doctor was shocked, he said, 'Did you get burned down there?' He couldn't recognise the circumcision. 'Eight months you were married and you were closed, maybe someone burned you and the thing is closed.'

Such comments sadly were common, as pointed out by the women. Every time they were confronted by such remarks, they felt humiliated and ashamed. One pointed out:

> They have to understand the physical and mental needs and the pain they went through. If the hospital, doctors or midwives when they see the private area and they get shocked and they give them a bad look, look surprised, this makes you feel worse, never comfortable with hospitals, so if they have problems they have to hide it, because she will know that person of care would be surprised, especially when a girl gets married they have to open again.

This was shown to be true and similar in a research conducted by Vangen et al.[12]

There is a need for the education of health professionals, especially in areas where there is a high prevalence of FGM women among its residents in the West.

They need to realise the sensitivity of this subject. As discussed by Vangen *et al.*,[12] Somali women found it difficult to express their concerns and fears openly, which led to a state of poor communication between both parties. Consequently, to prevent such a scenario from recurring, and as recommended by Vangen *et al.*,[12] the Royal College of Obstetricians and Gynaecologists[1] and the BMA,[13] the women should not be stigmatised and their fears should be addressed adequately by professionals who should attend to their needs.

A potential limitation of this study was the possible alteration to the essence of the conversations since they were translated to English from Arabic or Somali. Furthermore, time constraints did not permit independent corroboration of the themes, but they were deduced by closely following Boyatzis[4] methodology. Further validation through an independent rater is planned.

From this study, it was discovered that health professionals need to be made aware, educated and be able to enquire about FGM among women from high incidence areas during their consultations, without making them feel frightened or humiliated. Although health issues need to be discussed, the issue of the psychological effect of FGM on the woman's life should never be ignored. The practice of FGM is a harmful one, which affects women physically as well as psychologically.

A participant who was over 30 years of age was too traumatised to describe her experience of FGM; she broke down and cried on the remembrance of that day. Therefore support and counselling should always be offered if necessary. There is a great need for an extensive campaign about the health risks of FGM among women, as well as health professionals who may come across it. Most importantly, there is an urgent need for qualitative research into the psychological and medical effects of FGM on women, and the men's attitudes towards this practice.

A similar study to my own was conducted collaboratively by London Black Women's Health Action Project and the London School of Hygiene and Tropical Medicine in March of 1998. This involved in-depth interviews, as well as questionnaire-based analysis of the experiences, attitudes and the views of young, single Somalis on FGM, between the ages of 18–22 and living in London.[14] This study explored similar issues to this study, with the difference being that they concentrated their efforts on the single and young group of people in London, therefore there may be some discrepancies in the comparison between these two studies due to the groups' characteristics and place of residence.

In spite of these differences, the findings of both surveys have revealed that the vast majority of the women were FGM between the ages of 6–8 years, mostly of Type 3 infibulation, regardless of their place of birth. Interestingly, compared to my study, the majority of my participants were FGM at home (61%) regardless of their place of birth, including British-born participants; unlike this survey where all their British-born participants were FGM in a clinic/hospital by a doctor, nurse or midwife.

In terms of their attitudes, the same viewpoints were displayed in both studies in respect of the fact that some participants requested to FGM while others were surprised. The descriptions that were given here by these participants have echoed my own findings, for example the use of thorns, the pain, difficulty with urination and their menstrual cycle. Nevertheless, it was difficult to assess the impact of FGM on sexual function among my participants unlike this study, as my interview groups were mixed between the young and the old, the single and the married, and since premarital sexual activity is prohibited in Islam and the Somali culture, the single young girls who were not married will not admit to premarital sexual activity.

However, the general opinion among the consequences of FGM on sexual function was divided within my participants, as some said that it did not affect it since the only sexual partner they have had was their husbands so they don't know any different. Others said that FGM stopped them from enjoying their sexual pleasure, which was similar to the findings in this study where the participants agreed that FGM, especially infibulation, does affect your sexual function, largely due to the pain experienced.

The reasons that were given for the continuation of this practice were similar as well, with both studies showing that participants believed that religion, culture, preventing the woman from being dirty, and preventing the girl from being promiscuous were the reasons for this practice and its continuation. My study involved the opinions and attitudes of women towards FGM, and the men's attitudes were discovered from direct questioning of these female participants.

This study provided the missing link, whereby my participants said that some male supporters of FGM maintain their position, since they regard FGM to be part of the Somali tradition and Islamic practices, and a way of preserving honour to ensure the girl is wed, since a girl needs to be a virgin before marriage. A few others, especially the young men, prefer a girl not to be FGM. However, according to the above study, it was shown that young Somali men still believed and supported the reasons given above for this practice, and a third of them preferred to marry a girl who has undergone FGM. For those who opposed this practice, their reasons were that sexual satisfaction for both partners could not be achieved and the pain and sorrow that was caused by the de-infibulation procedure.

Finally, in terms of the recommendations for the way forward, both studies have shown that both groups have agreed that health and religious education about the consequences of this practice and the essence of such procedure needs to be highlighted in young and old, through education that might change attitudes and understanding of FGM.

I would like to thank the following people who helped and supported me during the study: Mr RW Stones, Dr Sandra Horne, Miss Karen Creed, my family, friends and all the participants.

References

1 Royal College of Obstetricians and Gynaecologists (2003) *Female Genital Mutilation: Statement No. 3*. RCOG, London.
2 World Health Organization (WHO 2000) *Female Genital Mutilation: Factsheet No. 241*. WHO, Geneva.
3 www.theodora.com/maps.
4 Boyatzis RE (1998) *Transforming qualitative information: Thematic analysis and code development*. Sage Publications, California.
5 Gibeau AM (1998) Female genital mutilation: when a cultural practice generates clinical and ethical dilemmas. *J Obstet Gynecol Neonatal Nurs.* **27**(1): 85–91.
6 Berry JW (1997) Immigration, acculturation and adaptation. *Applied psychology: An international review.* **46**(1): 5–68.
7 Cook RJ, Dickens BM and Fathalla MF (2002) Female genital cutting (mutilation/circumcision): ethical and legal dimensions. *Int J of Gynecol & Obstet.* **79**(3): 281–7.

8   Nour NM (2003) Female genital cutting: a need for reform. *Obstetrics and Gynaecology.* **101**(5)(Supplement): 1051–2.

9   Almroth L, Almroth-Berggren V, Hassanein OM *et al.* (2001) A community based study on the change of practice of female genital mutilation in a Sudanese village. *Int J of Gynecol and Obstet.* **74**(2): 179–85.

10 Nkwo PO and Onah HE (2001) Decrease in female genital mutilation among Nigerian Ibo girls. *Int J of Gynecol and Obstet.* **75**(3): 321–2.

11 Snow R (2001) Female genital cutting: distinguishing the rights from the health agenda. *Tropical Medicine and International Health.* **6**(2): 89.

12 Vangen SR, Johansen EB, Sundby J *et al.* (2004) Qualitative study of perinatal care experiences among Somali women and local health care professionals in Norway. *European Journal of Obstetrics and Gynaecology.* **112**(1): 29–35.

13 BMA (2001) *Female Genital Mutilation: Caring for patients and child protection.* British Medical Association, London.

14 Williams L, Dirir S, Warsame J, Dirir A, Elmi S (unpublished) *Experiences, attitudes and views of young, single Somalis living in London in Female Circumcision.*

Chapter Ten

Community development approaches: a case for female genital mutilation (FGM)

Sarah McCulloch

Introduction

This chapter explores how community development approaches (CDA) can be utilised to work in partnership with women and girls affected by the culturally sensitive and illegal practice of female genital mutilation (FGM). Before I can define and analyse what CDA is and how its approaches in theory and practice can be utilised to work with the culturally sensitive and illegal practice of female genital mutilation (FGM), also known as female circumcision (FC), I need to define what we mean by a 'community' and what 'development' involves. As Taylor noted,[1] defining a community is a complex issue, as any geographical community will include people whose primary identity is based on different factors, for example class, race, gender or sexual orientation. In this case the various communities that practise FGM are united by the gender and sexual orientation and yet are from all over Africa, Middle East and various parts of Asia and South America.[2]

How one defines a community is important because it influences the way one interacts with or views their needs, and how representatives are identified. Community development is a process of empowering and developing people in the local communities in which they live, but one might ask whether the community development approach can apply to an issue such as the culturally sensitive and secretive practice of FGM, which is never discussed or even mentioned by communities who practise it or by the girls and women affected by it.[3]

The principles underpinning a community development approach (CDA) are 'social justice, equity and democracy, working to foster community participation and empowerment, and development of partnerships'. The term has been used in a variety of undertakings and tends to be applied amongst vulnerable or disadvantaged communities to help in finding shared solutions to shared problems. People working together on important issues to the community to bring about change, empowerment, targeting of resources and optimal participation of target population in improving physical, psychological, socio-economic and environmental well-being, are considered amongst the best features of such an approach.

Its effective utilisation necessitates service providers possessing appropriate facilitation skills and a long-term commitment at strategic management level with regard to funding and other resource provision. It implies a process by which the efforts of the people themselves are united with those of government, and voluntary and other organisations to improve the community's circumstances and to integrate those communities into the life of the host nation.[4]

This process is made up of two essential elements: first, the participation by people themselves in efforts to improve their lives with as much reliance as possible on their own initiative; second, the provision of technical and other services, which encourage inventiveness, self-help and mutual support and make these more effective.

Thus community development is a means of working to stimulate and encourage communities to express their needs and to support them in their collective action, and involves working with community groups to identify their own health needs and concerns, and to take appropriate action.[5,6] Community development is also based on promoting a positive action approach to equal opportunities and encouraging people with the least power in society to gain more control over their lives. This involves the reallocation of resources to target the socially excluded, the integration of health within comprehensive social and economic regeneration and community participation in health planning.[4,7]

It starts with the community identifying priorities, and concepts of health based on holistic ideals, which are more broadly based than those imposed by external agencies and health workers.[2,8] In theory, community development aims to strengthen communities and improve their quality of life by releasing the potential within communities' 'added value', developing the skills, confidence and resources to address health problems and improve their welfare.[1,2,9] The aforementioned principles were based on the Alma Ata Declaration (1978) and 'Health For All' (HFA) and became the leading social models of community development and health promotion.[10]

Community development approaches in the UK

Community development in the UK emerged against the background of the welfare state and now operates in a much more open market, with current policies laying more emphasis on consumerism, participation, consultation and social inclusion.[13,14] Early community development approaches were to be found in the nineteenth century, when community workers helped the poor help themselves, providing skills and leadership in such initiatives as the Settlement Movement.[1,5]

Community development approaches gained momentum in the UK in the 1960s, drawing on colonial experiences after people returned from working with indigenous communities.[4] The Gulbenkian Foundation study in 1968 together with the Seebohm Report on personal and social services provided the impetus for the recognition of community development, as a distinctive approach.[1] In Britain the approach continued at a localised level with small-scale projects and organised support groups.

Major initiatives such as urban regeneration programmes and national community development projects were set up to seek new ways of tackling social problems, through local co-ordination of services and promoting self-help activities. This led to an increase in the employment of community workers in local authorities, with numbers reaching over 5000 in the mid 1980s.[13]

The word 'community' conveyed a sense of togetherness, of social cohesion and of releasing energies beyond those of each individual member.[8,14] Local authorities began to decentralise services and cultivate initiatives to benefit marginalised groups.[1,8] Central government's cuts in social funding put a squeeze on community development initiatives, as local authorities came under financial pressure to reduce community development programmes, which most affected areas concerned with ethnic minorities and marginalised groups.

The 1990s saw the return of community development activities, in particular with expansion and strengthening of community issues through the European Union.[13] With the New Labour Government came a shift in policy back to social issues, combating inequalities, an emphasis on quality, community involvement or participation and social inclusion;[8,12] new government initiatives are often accompanied by 'new' funding being made available for new ventures.

In Sheffield, for example, community development activities operate on an informal level with groups with common interests and concerns; such groups include Refugee Lifeline, Communities Health Forum (CHF), Somali Special Needs Project (SSNP), Black Health Forum (BHF) and Agency for Culture and Change Management (ACCM).

In 1997, Sheffield Health Authority (SHA) produced *Involving the Public: A Strategy for Community Development*, which highlighted SHA's clear understanding of the diverse communities and their perceived needs and values and how these relate to health and well-being; the empowerment of communities to reduce inequalities in health and to promote shared working and partnership.

Criticisms of community development approaches

Community development approaches have been criticised from all sides, including by marginalised groups themselves. They have been criticised for not challenging inequalities based on ethnicity or gender and for creating class formation in deprived areas, which extends and deepens the patterns of inequality and intensifies competition for scarce resources of all kinds.[4,8]

Women's groups have argued that community development focuses on class inequalities and interests and tends to overlook gender divisions and conflicts, with gender inequalities being considered secondary to class or ethnic inequalities. Many have argued that women and other marginalised groups hardly get consulted; colonial records on African 'traditions' were exclusively derived from male informants and indigenous female beliefs remained unrecorded. This may explain why FGM has remained a secret custom for so long because the men – who are often excluded – have been the ones interviewed about FGM.[15]

There is a tendency for employers or sponsors to see community development programmes as time-consuming, concentrating on small numbers of people and using large resources for the sake of dubious results which could not be quantified, such as inequalities or lack of access to health services.[1,6] Previous experiences in Britain have also demonstrated that it is perceived as an overtly political strategy.

The political implications of community development have been attacked from both the left and right wings of the political spectrum. It is viewed on the one hand as a subversive left-wing activity; and on the other, as a subtle means of policing and controlling communities by socialists.[8] This latter view would summarise the community development programmes in Third World countries where community development initiatives were not seen as ideas from the communities themselves, but those imposed by colonial administrators for the benefit of colonial interests; the poor section of the community received little gain.[4,16]

The objective of working on the community's own terms and priority issues fails to deliver. With reference to FGM programmes in the UK since 1985, and in Africa since colonisation there seems to be no evidence that any real change has taken place, despite community development programmes being in operation for over 50 years in the case of Sudan. The practice is still continuing, though there is something to be said for the awareness raised so far that has led to some change in attitudes in some communities. For example, Somalis now talk about being in favour of performing the milder Type 1 Sunna and not the brutal infibulation.[17]

The other problem with community development approaches is its assumption that the community is homogeneous with shared common interests; however, a community is complex and riddled with conflict. The Somali community, for example, is full of complexities, beset with tribal and gender-related problems, not to mention the issue of FGM, which is little understood.[9,18] These factors serve to undermine the assumptions and aims of community development approaches.

Evaluation of community development approaches to FGM

There are various health promotion/education and community care programmes within countries that practise FGM, many of which have been organised and financed by non-governmental organisations (NGOs), United Nations (UN), World Health Organization (WHO), United Nations International Children's Emergency Fund (UNICEF), Amnesty International (AI) and various other organisations with an interest in health and the welfare of girls and women. The majority of these programmes are based on community development approaches, which involve the communities themselves through empowerment initiatives.

We should not underestimate work being done by smaller local community groups or individuals, who are striving to get the message against FGM across to their communities, such as the Sudanese National Committee and the National Council for Women in Kenya. There is also an African umbrella organisation covering Africa, the Inter-African Committee on Traditional Practices (IAC) based in Geneva with offices in Sudan, Kenya and Senegal. The IAC often holds symposia, conferences and meetings to keep FGM issues on the agenda and campaign towards its eradication.

In Somalia, the Somali Women's Democratic Organization (SWDO) set up in 1977 by the then government is still campaigning, although this is on a low-key basis due to lack of funding and strong opposition from the community. New programmes being set up by BWHFS and led by Shamis Dirie may precipitate more activity with funding support from overseas organisations and governments.

In West and South Yorkshire, The Agency for Culture and Change Management (ACCM) is the major campaigner. A small local descriptive study based on needs assessment sought to evaluate to what extent community development objectives were being met in improving access to health service provision for FGM victims from the local Somali community. Descriptive research methodology requires extensive background knowledge of the situation or community, so that one knows appropriate aspects on which to gather information and I drew on my previous five years of work with the Somali community.

The study involved collection, analysis and interpretation of data from open structured questionnaire on knowledge of FGM and ACCM, existing health problems, health services or programmes, constraints or problems, social stratification, focal points of resistance or high prevalence. Qualitative and quantitative techniques included questionnaires, interviews, observation of participants, service statistics and documents describing communities, FGM practices, groups, situations, programmes or services and other individual or ecological units.[19,20]

The process was interactive, person to person, to establish meanings and clear understandings, which have many implications; one of them being that the process actually changes people, including the people undertaking the research.[20] The purpose of the study was to gather empirical data, which the focus group approach had failed to provide, and to establish the views of a selected number of members of the Somali community.

I selected participants and interviewed the eight women and four men. Access to them was not a problem, but interviewing venues had to be agreed in advance. Two questionnaires were used, one for the women and one for the men, and they were composed of a mixture of open-ended and structured questions to enable me to explore issues and provide relevant information on the Somali community's attitudes, beliefs, fears about FGM, ACCM and its work and the health services.

Methodology provided simple, straightforward information on attitudes, motives, values and beliefs in relation to FGM. It is adaptable and the interviewer had the opportunity to probe further for more information or clarify issues not made clear or understood by the interviewee. It allows the interviewer to reassure the interviewee of the confidentiality and anonymity of the interview and ensure support for the research, as Somalis are generally unwilling to discuss FGM openly. Due to the secretive and sensitive nature of the practice, tape recording was not allowed, as no one wished to leave any evidence that would later identify participants; hence use of coding.

Assurances were given that codes were to be used to maintain anonymity in the interviews and report and this guarantee was enforced by the fact that a draft report would be made available to them for approval before it was submitted. This ensured trust and confidence in those who agreed to be interviewed. This was most important, as it was felt that some of the information was personal and might damage the standing of those involved and lead to their being stigmatised or rejected by their community.

I personally regard the maintenance of confidentiality and anonymity for the respondents as an issue of professional and personal integrity. I did not wish to be seen to be betraying the community or the respondents for the benefit of the organisation I work for or myself. ACCM funded the study and any information and knowledge gained will be utilised in my work and to improve the services ACCM are providing on issues relating to FGM.

Questionnaires had four main sections. The first was about the work of ACCM, the second about participants, the third on the issue of FGM and the fourth on health services. For the purposes of this chapter, study findings and conclusions are summarised and mainly drawn from Sections 1 and 4.

Community development work by ACCM

Section 1 analysed the responses and views of respondents on the existence of ACCM, approaches being used in its work, its management committee and staff and what they wanted ACCM to do. The results were presented in numbers and percentages with graphics to illustrate responses. No inferential tests of statistical significance have been undertaken due to the small size of the sample (n = 12).

Asked if they had heard about ACCM and its work, 83% said 'yes', while 17% said 'no'. Asked how they had heard about ACCM, 50% said they heard from staff, 17% from a member of the management committee and 33% heard from members of the Somali community. 83% said they had heard 'a lot of rumours', most of them hostile, about the project.

This did not surprise me, as word spreads round the Somali community very quickly, especially if it is something they are unhappy about. People process information in many ways once they have been exposed to it; they can either respond positively by being involved or negatively by peripheral information processing, which lacks the active awareness, comprehension and evaluation of arguments to support their position.[21]

The majority commented that the only way forward is to involve the community but at the same time they contradicted themselves by adding that the issues are too sensitive and the community do not talk about it. This finding is similar to that of other researchers who all agree that the community needs to be consulted but that the issues are difficult to bring out into the open, as communities do not readily disclose information.[2,9,18,22]

Only two male and one female respondents spoke strongly about wanting the practice of FGM eliminated by the Agency, but stressed it has to be done gradually over time and through education. Comments made in favour of FGM included:

> Why should it stop just because we live in Sheffield? This is our culture and has been going on for centuries.
>
> > Female respondent
>
> My grandmother did it to my mother, my mother did it to me and I will do it to my daughter.
>
> > Female respondent
>
> If I don't do it who will marry my daughters?
>
> > Female respondent
>
> It is a good thing for them, women, it stops them flirting.
>
> > Male respondent

Those who were against it said that it was too painful and that they could not justify putting their daughters through it and it was risky. As one commented:

> ...all that blood and pain, no I would not have my future children go through it. This practice is for old people in villages in Somalia ...

Asked whether there were alternatives to initiating girls instead of the painful practice, the majority (91% — 10 out of 11) of respondents said education was the main alternative. If girls get the education then they will get jobs and there will be no need for FGM. As one female and one male commented:

> They do not do it in Saudi Arabia or Iran, very strong Muslim countries, why do we do it?

One male respondent was sceptical about any chances of eliminating this practice,

> ... this thing is done by women on women, it is their secret, they never talk to any one about it, men have no say in it, who is going to convince them to stop especially those back in Somalia in the villages? I don't know ... wait and see ... it will take a long time ...

Legal issues

Asked if they were aware that FGM was illegal in the UK and in some African countries, 25% of female respondents said they knew FGM was illegal in the UK, while 50% said they didn't know FGM was illegal. Only one male respondent was aware of the legal implications of FGM in the UK and in some African countries. This is worrying, considering that FGM has been illegal since 1985, when many Somalis were already residing in the UK but could be explained by the fact that many Somalis are illiterate.[23]

Health services

Section 4 was concerned with finding out what health services are used, what is available and what other services the Somali community needs which are currently not available. This section also aimed to discover whether girls or women have been treated differently because they were circumcised.

Asked which health services they knew about, the majority listed hospitals, general practitioners (GPs), health visitors (HVs) and physiotherapists. One mentioned community care/carer services and community midwives. Asked which services they used most, GPs, hospitals and HVs were again mentioned most. In addition, female respondents with children said they also made use of community health centres and Somali community groups such as the Isracc and The East African Women's Project in Darnal.

Asked if they felt they have been treated differently because they were circumcised, 55% of the women said 'yes', 36% said 'no', with 9% saying they did not remember or did not know. In total, 36% said that their GPs or midwives had treated them differently during childbirth. The main reasons given were that GPs or other health professionals had no idea of FGM issues, never listened and often ignored what the patient was saying. One commented:

> ... you get treated like you are an 'alien' and that you are wasting their time.

All respondents said that, after the interview, they now understood more about FGM, and now appreciated the difficult work the agency was doing. Community development and health promotion approaches were seen as best in highlighting and raising awareness of health problems and in getting reluctant Somali women to listen and get help. It is less provocative, and is sensitive and easy to get people involved. Eliminating FGM will take time; there is potential to help girls and women face the facts that FGM has harmed their health and that they need help.

There is a need to keep raising awareness of legal issues and information should be presented in languages best understood by the local community. Professionals must be educated to understand and support the community in a sensitive way. It could be argued that those undermining ACCM's work are only extremists. The current hostility against ACCM will take time to dissolve, and as one respondent commented:

> Really all you need to do is to shout louder, raise awareness, provide the necessary information, education, improve access to services, make people more culturally sensitive and understanding of FGM issues to help those who are victims and prevent new cases.

Conclusion and recommendations

The study has attempted to assess whether community development approaches work in practice in relation to the work of ACCM on FGM issues. It examined the attitudes, characteristics and beliefs of the local Somali community, the largest FGM-practising community in Sheffield. The findings highlighted the success of using community development approaches but have also revealed the limitations.

To a certain degree and having conducted the study, I have changed my attitudes towards FGM. Although I feel it is child abuse in the extreme, I have accepted that it is their culture and any approach used to tackle it has to involve parents and to a large extent the community. ACCM's community development approaches seem ideal to tackle this sensitive issue but they are not enough, as the personality and characteristics of ACCM's workers play an important role in achieving access and dialogue that is acceptable for a hostile community that does not wish to discuss the issue or divulge any information.

I was fortunate in being able to access the Somali community and, because I am not Somali, this enabled respondents to discuss FGM issues openly. I was not perceived as a threat and would not stigmatise them, and also the community knew me from my previous work, as someone they could work with. This proved crucial when recruiting respondents for interview and being able to collect reliable information for the study.

The study highlighted the difficulty of using a community or a group, as a way to consult or involve the community on an issue of concern to them; FGM is seen as a personal issue and rarely discussed openly. The findings showed that community development approaches are, to a certain extent, appropriate for tackling FGM issues.

Community development approaches are based on long-term strategies that take into account other factors that affect the community and the individual. Such aims and objectives as health promotion and education, advocacy, providing relevant information and involving the party(ies) in the plans and implementing of agreed strategies are important, leading to empowerment of individuals and the community to take control of their lives.

During the study, information was provided to respondents during and after the interview. Even those who refused to acknowledge that they had health problems have since sought medical help from their doctors or health visitors. The information is being shared in the community through word of mouth and the publicity leaflets in Somali that ACCM has made available to the community. The issue of most significance to the community is the legal position, as the study showed that over 63% were not aware of the legal implications of FGM.

While some of the communities who practise FGM remain hostile to any work being undertaken to tackle FGM, they are now more responsive and wish to be involved as individuals, albeit secretively for fear of being stigmatised or rejected by the community. Community workers should tackle FGM by targeting individuals, who can then spread the message within their communities.

As other authors in this book have acknowledged, progress is very slow and it takes time for such a deeply rooted and sensitive practice to be eradicated. However, community development approaches can contribute to empowering the community to enable them to improve their quality of life and health and well-being, as much as possible through their own initiative, with workers and organisations providing that needed support when required.

Although the study found evidence that community development approaches can work in practice, the study also confirmed the complexities of dealing with the Somali community, with origins in Somalia, and who have immigrated with their tribal or clan beliefs and values intact and which are still strongly upheld in Sheffield.

Somali women do not see FGM as a health problem, and often reply to any concerns about their health with, 'We have done this for centuries with no problem, so why stop now?' They see housing, money, employment and racism – especially over health and education – as their main problems, not FGM. There is also a problem of inter-agency collaboration on FGM issues; some of the organisations in the UK see FGM as a cultural issue for those communities to deal with and that outside agencies should not interfere.

At the same time the same organisations are quick to pick up the legal issue that FGM is child abuse and needs to be stopped. These views have caused conflict between the agencies such as ACCM, statutory organisations like the police, health and child protection units and the community who resent interference of 'racist' organisations or individuals in their culture. It is a stark truth that there is little or no consensus on how to approach FGM issues and for as long as this situation continues, the practice will persist.

References

1   Taylor M (1988) *Signposts to Community Development*. Community Development Foundation, London.
2   World Health Organization (1996) *Female Genital Mutilation: A Joint WHO/UNICEF/UNFPA Statement*. WHO, Geneva.
3   Smithies J and Adams L (1990) *Community Participation In Health Promotion*. London Health Education Authority, London.
4   McPherson S (1982) *Social Policy in the Third World. The Social Dilemmas of Underdevelopment*. Wheatsheaf Books Ltd, Brighton.
5   Oakley P (1989) *Community Involvement in Health Development: An examination of the critical issues*. World Health Organization, Geneva.
6   Ewles L and Simnett I (1992) *Promoting Health: A Practical Guide*. Scutari Press, London.

7   Djukanovic V and Mach EP (1975) *Alternative Approaches to Meeting Basic Health Needs in Developing Countries.* WHO, Geneva.

8   Naidoo J and Wills J (1994) *Health Promotion: Foundation for Practice.* Baillière Tindall, Edinburgh.

9   Dorkenoo E (1995) *Cutting the Rose. Female genital mutilation: the practice and its prevention.* Minority Rights Publications, London.

10 World Health Organization (1987) *Evaluation of the Strategy for Health For All by Year 2000. 7th Report of the World Health Situation.* WHO, Geneva.

11 Department of Health (1992) *The Health of The Nation Strategy for the Health of England.* DoH, London.

12 Department of Health (1998) *Health of The Nation Consultation Document.* DoH, London.

13 McConnell C (1991) *Promoting Community Development in Europe: Research and Policy Paper No. 15.* Community Development Foundation, London.

14 Wilkinson RG (1996) *Unhealthy Societies: the afflictions of inequality.* Routledge, London.

15 Hobsbawm E and Ranger T (1993) *The Invention of Tradition.* Cambridge University Press, Cambridge.

16 Dore R and Mars Z (1981) *Community Development: comparative case studies in India, The Republic of Korea, Mexico and Tanzania.* Croom Helm, London.

17 Dirie W and Miller C (1999) Desert Flower. *The Reader's Digest.* **10**: 136–61.

18 Walker A (1993) *Warrior Marks: female genital mutilation and the sexual blinding of women.* Harcourt Brace, Florida.

19 Miles M and Huberman A (1994) *Qualitative Data Analysis: an expanded sourcebook* (2e). Sage Publications, London.

20 Norton P and Stewart M (1991) *Primary Care Research: traditional and innovative approaches 1.* Sage, London.

21 Maibach E and Parrott RL (1995) *Designing Health Messages: approaches from communication theory and public health practice.* Sage Publications Ltd., London.

22 Koso-Thomas O (1987) *The Circumcision of Women: a strategy for eradication.* ZED Books, London.

23 The Guardian (2000) The Right to Education. *The Guardian.* **28 February**: 15–16.

Chapter Eleven

Legislative action to eradicate FGM in the UK

Sadiya Mohammad

Introduction

Over the past three or four decades, FGM has increasingly emerged amongst ethnic minority groups in many countries, including the United Kingdom. This increase has been contemporaneous with the arrival of immigrants, economic migrants, asylum seekers, refugees and students from FGM-practising countries (such as Somalia, Sudan, Djibouti, Nigeria, Eritrea, Ethiopia and Sierra Leone). The 1985 Prohibition of Female Circumcision Act made FGM illegal in the UK, except on specific physical and mental health grounds. This Act was replaced by the Female Genital Mutilation Act 2003, which came into force on 3 March 2004.

Passing anti-FGM legislation has been one of the most controversial aspects of the campaign to stop FGM. The new law has been seen by many as a force which will bring us closer to eradicating the practice entirely. On the other hand, it has been argued that legislation against FGM, without robust political commitment and other proactive interventions, renders such legislation meaningless and even harmful. This chapter will explore these issues in more depth to discern the efficacy of legislative action in the elimination of FGM in the UK.

Methodology

The methodology formulated to carry out this research has been an exploratory two-phase process including:

- an extensive literature review and
- collection of qualitative data using focus group discussions and in-depth interviews.

The first phase involved an extensive review of both published and grey literature pertaining to FGM. This review has formed the basis of the knowledge needed to fully examine the practice of FGM both in the UK and abroad. It involved a thorough examination of the specific legislation on FGM in the UK, as well as the current approaches and strategies, which are used to address FGM.

The second phase consisted of the collection of qualitative data on FGM using in-depth interviews with key actors participating in the FGM discourse and members of the practising communities. This phase also included one focus group with several young Somali women, to gain greater insight into their feelings, beliefs and attitudes on FGM in the UK, and about anti-FGM laws.

The limitation of this method was the time frame and, as such, the inability to conduct a second focus group to count as a 'control'. Nevertheless, this phase was crucial in drawing on the wealth of experience from various bodies and their views on the possible strategies and policies that must be ensured for the elimination of FGM.

Female genital mutilation in the UK

Current situation in the UK: prevalence and distribution

During the past three or four decades, female circumcision has emerged in the UK, contemporaneous with the arrival of people from FGM-practising countries (such as Somalia, Sudan, Djibouti, Nigeria, Eritrea, Ethiopia and Sierra Leone) as economic migrants, asylum seekers, refugees or students.[1] The two most common forms of mutilation seen in the UK are type II and type III, and the main communities who practise it are from Eritrea, Ethiopia, Somalia and the Yemen.[2] In the UK, FGM is obtained in several ways. Families may know health professionals or traditional excisers who can carry out the procedure in the UK. It is not uncommon, however, for families to save money over long periods of time and take the girl abroad to undergo FGM.[3]

It is very difficult to get exact figures for genitally mutilated females or those 'at risk' of mutilation, as there have been no comprehensive surveys of the prevalence in the UK. Such studies are difficult, due to the secretive nature of the practice and the fact that communities that are likely to practise it are often marginalised and 'closed'.[4] Furthermore, the African population in the UK are relatively understudied, and are frequently homogenised under the category of 'Black' or 'African-Caribbean'.

The decennial census carried out in the UK fails to differentiate specifically between ethnic groups, with categories of 'black African/black British African', and thus classifies 53 potential African countries in one group.[5] Moreover, this position compounds the absence of any mandatory requirements or databases to monitor or record cases of FGM when they come to the attention of hospitals and other professionals.

Notwithstanding these difficulties, estimates have been provided by FOR-WARD using data figures from various studies and Home Office statistics on the numbers of immigrants, refugees and asylum applications from countries where FGM is endemic.[5] It is estimated that approximately 74 000 women in the UK have undergone FGM, and 7000 females are at risk of genital mutilation every year.[6]

Why does FGM persist in the UK?

It has been argued that where FGM is near ubiquitous, in countries in Africa for example, women living in these countries have very limited spheres, as they are surrounded by the practice. A direct corollary of this is the inability to compare their condition with that of women who have not been genitally mutilated.[7] In the

UK, where FGM is not widespread, and it is seen by many as largely 'unacceptable', one may assume that practising communities are more likely to relinquish such practices in the pursuit of acculturation. However, this has not been the case.

Empirical evidence suggests that people that move to a new country generally take their traditions and customs with them. Many ethnic groups practising FGM in the UK live in very tight-knit communities and acculturation into their host country rarely occurs. The desire to romanticise and hold on to their cultural identity is naturally very strong in a new and sometimes alien culture.[4] As a result, many families may buttress FGM, as a form of social control; ensuring children do not lose ties with their traditional society. FGM, in this context, becomes a mechanism preventing the girl from masturbating, engaging in sexual intercourse and otherwise being drawn into what may be perceived as a decadent British culture.

Legislative developments in the UK

Human rites vs human rights

In the UK, FGM is regarded as a form of child abuse.[8] However, it differs from other forms of abuse, in that it is done with the best intentions for the future welfare of the child, it is not repeated during childhood and it is widely accepted by the sections of the communities in which it is practised.

> Human behaviours and cultural values, however senseless or destructive they may look to us from our particular personal and cultural standpoints, have meaning and fulfil a function for those who practise them.
> Statement by WHO Director General to
> 1994 Global Commission on Women's Health[9]

In the UK, FGM presents a 'cross-cultural problem' encompassing a practice which is viewed as acceptable within the culture it occurs, but as abusive and harmful by others.[10] As such, criticisms of the practice, which are deeply embedded in culture and tradition, can be seen as highly controversial, or even racist, and seen as criticisms of the culture and tradition in its entirety. It is not surprising therefore that when FGM first emerged in the UK, a *laissez faire* attitude was taken, rooted in the belief that cultures should be left to develop and change at their own pace, free from external influence.[11]

This idea of 'cultural relativism' *a propos* FGM has been challenged by many human rights activists, who maintain that cultures should only be sacrosanct insofar as they are in line with human rights.

Cultural claims cannot be invoked to justify their violation (human rights) and those that argue against FGM on human rights grounds cannot be accused of making non-imperialist attacks on culture.[12]

The human rights implications of FGM have been unequivocally recognised at the international level, as rights which are universal and that transcend cultures and societies. As such, several conventions[6] specifically addressing FGM as 'violation of human rights', 'violence against women' and 'child abuse' have been formulated and widely ratified.

Medicalisation of FGM

FGM attracted media attention in the early 1980s, not because of its historical presence or due to the inflow of migrants from certain African ethnic groups, but because it became known that private clinics in London were performing FGM for women and girls coming from overseas. The business was mainly from African elites and thus offered massive economic benefits to these clinics.[5]

In the ensuing debate, some argued that as such procedures could carry such dire health outcomes it would be better if performed in sterile conditions, by qualified personnel and under anaesthetic.[13] Anti-FGM activists strongly disagree with such propositions, as do many international medical associations, on human rights grounds. The World Health Organization (WHO) has endorsed this view:

> Medicalisation of the procedure does not eliminate this harm (FGM) and is inappropriate for two major reasons: genital mutilation runs against basic ethics of health care, and its medicalisation seems to legitimise the harmful practice.[14]

The WHO has consistently and unequivocally advised that FGM should not be practised by any health professional in any setting. This position has been met with near-universal consensus by international agencies and NGOs, asserting that no action will entrench FGM more than legitimating it through the medical profession.[15] It has also been argued that as FGM is a human rights issue, the protection of these rights must be under the auspices of the British Government. It was this continuous lobbying from NGOs and other agencies, which provided the major impetus for the UK Government to pass the first law in 1985 prohibiting female circumcision.

> No cultural, medical or other reason can ever justify a practice that causes so much pain and suffering. Regardless of cultural background, it is completely unacceptable and should be illegal wherever it takes place.[16]

Prohibition of Female Circumcision Act 1985

The Prohibition of Female Circumcision Act 1985 made genital mutilation illegal in the UK. Section 1(1) of the Act stated that it shall be an offence for any person:

a   To excise, infibulate or otherwise mutilate the whole or any part of the labia majora or labia minora or clitoris of another person; or
b   To aid, alert, counsel, or procure the performance by another person of any of those acts on that other person's own body.

The consequent penalties are:

c   On conviction or indictment, a fine or imprisonment not exceeding five years or to both; or
d   On summary conviction, to a fine not exceeding the statutory maximum or to imprisonment for a term not exceeding six months, or both.

This Act prevented medical professionals carrying out the procedures and also made it illegal for re-infibulation to be carried out following childbirth. Section 2 of the Act, however, provides an exemption if such procedures are necessary for the physical or mental health of person. It was thus permissible to carry out procedures in connection with childbirth, for gender reassignment and cosmetic surgery, if performed by a qualified health professional. Although there was no clarification of what constitutes 'mental health grounds', it explicitly states that no account is taken of any cultural beliefs, traditions or rituals which demand the practice.[5]

Despite substantial evidence of the practice occurring in the UK, there have been no successful prosecutions under the 1985 Act, and FGM in the UK has continued largely unabated. Practising communities living in Britain have held on strongly to their cultural beliefs, and despite the legislation have continued the practice either illegally in the UK, or abroad. Many families can circumvent the 1985 Act by taking children abroad temporarily to be circumcised.[17]

Closing this loophole has been a move supported for years by anti-FGM campaigners and a recommendation of an All Party Parliamentary Group on Population, Development and Reproductive Health, reporting in 2000.[18] Other recommendations included raising awareness among practising communities on legislation against FGM, and other measures to accelerate the elimination of FGM in the UK. Christine McCafferty, chair of the cross-party group, declared that 'it is not only unacceptable that there have been no prosecutions for female genital mutilation under the UK law of 1985, but that awareness of the law is minimal'.[19]

The Female Genital Mutilation Act 2003

In view of recommendations to close the loophole in the 1985 Act, which allowed girls to be taken abroad and circumcised, a Private Members Bill was introduced by Ann Clwyd MP in 2003, and came into force on 3 March 2004. The Female Genital Mutilation Act 2003 repeals and re-enacts the 1985 Act.

The 2003 Act has a number of benefits over its predecessor:

- First, the title of the Act describes more accurately the prohibited acts and acknowledges the practice as an act of mutilation. This removes any suggestion of acceptability that the word 'circumcision' might imply.[17]
- Second, the law gives extraterritorial effect to the existing provisions, and thus closes the loophole of the 1985 Act. For the first time, it is an offence for a UK national or permanent UK resident to carry out FGM abroad, or to aid, abet, counsel or procure the carrying out of FGM abroad, even in countries where the practice may be legal.
- Third, the Act increases the maximum penalty for performing and procuring FGM from 5 to 14 years imprisonment.

The issue of legislating against FGM is very complex, and ratification of the FGM Act 2003 has raised several questions. How will this new law be enforced? Will it be any more effective than the 1985 Act? What needs to be done to ensure that such a law is effective? How can legislation be used, as an effective tool for the elimination of FGM?

Perception of legislative action against FGM

Passing anti-FGM legislation has been one of the most controversial aspects of the FGM elimination movement. On the one hand, the new law has been seen by many as a force which will bring us closer to eradicating FGM entirely.[16] On the other, it has been argued that legislation against FGM, without robust political commitment and other proactive interventions (media campaigns, community education and empowerment programmes), leaves such legislation as meaningless.

Advantages of legislating against FGM

In the main, activists and analysts have maintained that one of the important advantages of legislating against FGM is that it provides an official platform to back up their positions by empowering them with the necessary legal support. Moreover, it gives the relevant authorities (health professionals, police, social workers) the legitimacy to intervene, and 'makes them brave enough to come forward without fear that they are being racist or culturally insensitive'.[16]

In an interview with Comfort Momoh, a specialist midwife on FGM, she stated that such legislation was important in the UK, as it gave health professionals an official reason for rejecting the medicalisation of the practice and for refusing to comply with demands for re-infibulation after delivery.[20] In addition, a law means that members of the practising communities who do not want to carry out FGM on their girls can invoke the law to back up their position. The sanctions of the law may also act as a deterrent to those who may want to continue the practice, but fear prosecution.[21]

Boyles and Preves contend that 'laws have real consequences in fuelling eradication efforts, regardless of whether local individuals are actually prosecuted under them'.[22] Therefore the legislation against FGM is necessary in demonstrating to society that the practice is a violation of human rights and will not be tolerated by the state.[11] If enforced correctly it could work to increase awareness by the general public and practising communities on FGM and its consequences. It could also lead to an increase in resources for organisations and agencies working towards the elimination of FGM.

Disadvantages and scepticism over anti-FGM laws

It has been argued that by only changing the law, the 'government has concentrated on the recommendation that has cost them nothing'.[21] In this context, the old axiom, 'changing the law is easier than changing society' is apposite. The regulatory role of the law has been recognised; however, what is less apparent is whether the law is an appropriate tool in tackling a practice like FGM, so deeply ingrained in culture. Difficulties in enforcing the law and adverse effects it may have on practising communities are points that have been frequently cited by critics.

Many FGM activists have remained sceptical of the prospective efficacy of the new law against FGM. The agnosticism is partly the result of the shortcomings of the 1985 law, failing to prosecute any perpetrators of FGM. Thus illustrating the existence of a law does not necessarily lead to its subsequent enforcement. Furthermore, a law will not change traditions and customs that have been in existence for centuries.

This was reflected in the views of several young Somali men and women living in London. A survey commissioned by the Department of Health in 1998 found that 42% of males and 18% of females from this community had intentions of circumcising their own daughters irrespective of prohibitive legislation. In interviews with Somali women in London, many supported this view, stating that although the law was an important initiative: 'Somalis hold on so tightly to the culture they have been brought up with, and the respect for the culture will be much greater than the respect for a law.'[23]

Another concern is the difficulty in identifying females that might be at risk of FGM and the lack of protocols for reporting any suspected cases. In tight-knit communities where FGM is practised, members hold on very strongly to traditions and community values, and are unlikely to betray one another to the law. Once FGM has been performed, the female does not necessarily face continuing risk, and the secret nature of the practice also makes it increasingly challenging to identify what child may be at risk. These challenges are increased by the juxtaposition of a culture, which restricts girls from discussing FGM openly and the rarity of routine examination of a girl's genitalia.

In a survey carried out in 2000, only 46% of organisations that play a key role in FGM policies (including health and social services, NGOs, education authorities and refugee councils) mentioned an awareness of the 1985 Act.[24] The lack of awareness of legislation against FGM, and the fear of being thought of as racist or culturally insensitive, are reasons often cited by health professionals and other authorities on why they do not report many FGM cases. Moreover, the powers that children have under the Act to refuse examination, and the difficulty of establishing in a court that a child is at risk of abuse, explains some of the difficulties that relevant authorities are likely to face in enforcing the new legislation.

One of the frequently mentioned apprehensions pertaining to anti-FGM laws is the possibility that such action has driven the practice underground. As a result, legislative action against FGM may work to vitiate several FGM elimination strategies based on community participation, as the trust for health professionals and NGOs may be reduced. As a direct corollary of this, activists and health professionals fear that they may be up against a 'wall of silence', as people may be less likely to come forward and share their experiences of FGM.[25]

Additionally, the health needs of women who have undergone FGM, including complications associated with the practice, may go unnotified for fear of the repercussions to their families. This leaves many FGM sufferers without access to essential medical services, and results in poor evidence-based strategies for dealing with and eliminating FGM.

It has been acknowledged that the law is only one component to the solution of the FGM problem. Baroness Scotland, the Minister of State for the criminal justice system and law, has clearly stated that:

> Law on its own will not stop it (FGM), it's just one of the ingredients that we need to have to make sure the change that we aspire to happen actually takes place.[14]

Adwoa Kwateng-Kluvitse, the director of FORWARD, has maintained that the best approach needed to effectively address FGM in the UK is for the enactment of the law to go hand-in-hand with community education and robust commitment from the government.[21]

Ways forward

Although the formulation of the 2003 Act provides a strong foundation to support and sustain the ongoing work of activists and NGOs in the fight against FGM, it has become quite apparent that legislation alone will not eradicate the practice. To properly address the problem of FGM in the UK, a number of factors need to be addressed. These will include training of professionals on FGM, robust political commitment and education and empowerment of women and communities.

Training for professionals

Due to the frequency that health professionals and statutory sector professionals are in contact with FGM-practising communities, they are likely to be the first to discover cases of FGM. However, they are often reluctant to address such cases, for fear that they might be perceived as racist or culturally insensitive. Moreover, the fact that the nature of the practice is intricately located within a sexual and reproductive sphere, making it 'taboo' in many cultures, means that women are often disinclined to talk about their experiences.[26]

These compounding factors have made FGM increasingly convenient to ignore. However, health professionals and other relevant authorities (including social services, the education system and the police force) are in the best position to recognise and monitor cases of FGM, and thus identify females that may be at risk of the practice. As such, their role is critical in enforcing the new legislation.

A number of medical organisations have published guidelines and position papers on the issue of FGM. These include Royal College of Nursing,[27] the Royal College of Midwives,[28] Royal College of General Practitioners[29] and the British Medical Association.[2,30] These papers and guidelines were issued to emphasise the need for healthcare professionals (HCPs) to know about the health and legal issues surrounding FGM. Moreover, the papers were intended to disseminate information; not only to HCPs, but also to the communities they serve. Additionally, they played a part in highlighting that FGM was unacceptable and that the respective organisation had a part to play in its prevention.

> Where doctors come across this kind of mutilation (FGM), they have a duty to take actions in reporting it.[16]

HCPs have an important contribution to make through the provision of health information and health promotion. They can raise awareness of the harmful effects of FGM amongst the general public, other medical professionals, decision-makers (including Government members) and the communities where FGM is widespread. They thus need to be aware of at-risk groups and need to suspect that any woman from the countries where FGM is practised is likely to have undergone genital mutilation. For example, if an infibulated woman gives birth, after delivery the midwife should inform the health visitor who takes over the care of the baby for the following five years.[21]

It is important for the health visitor to continue with the education of the woman as, if the mother has undergone FGM, it is likely that that the child might also be subjected to FGM. If a girl is suspected to be at risk of FGM, the HCP caring for her has a duty to ensure that there is a dialogue with the family concerning the health and legal risks of carrying out such an act.[2]

They also have a responsibility in enforcing the current law on FGM by notifying the correct authority, social service child protection units, for example. The right to confidentiality and parents' rights to autonomy are vitiated, when breaching these rights may be necessary to protect a child from serious harm.[31] Although the new legislation provides social service departments with the necessary legal backing to properly investigate cases of FGM, and deal with such cases appropriately, the first step must be to inform and educate the families and communities, and the law should only be used as a last resort.

Rahmat Mohammad, an FGM activist working with FORWARD, warned:

> We don't want a law which is used to remove the child from their parents; we want to be able to support the parents so they will protect their own children.[32]

Many FGM-practising communities in the UK view social workers as agents that 'take children away from families and [agents that are] insensitive to the cultural beliefs and traditions of that family'.[25] This fear of being seen as insensitive to other traditions and cultures has resulted in very few notifications of FGM cases. Critics have contended that this failure to pursue a course of action for fear of antagonism in that community is in its own way a form of racism, in that 'it is a retreat based on racial considerations to the detriment of the child'.[1]

The physical and psychological complications of FGM can have detrimental effects on the school life of many adolescent girls. Studies have shown that tightly infibulated girls may spend much longer in school toilets due to difficulties in voiding.

In an interview with an infibulated Somali student living in London, she pointed out the distress regarding her time at secondary school. She was 'frequently absent from school due to abdominal pains, and heavy menstruation', and did not feel that she was able to approach any of her teachers for fear of being looked upon as a 'freak' or of 'judgements passed on (her) culture'.[26] Even when schools are aware of the conditions of their pupils, there is often a 'culture of silence', which prevails. This is compounded by the lack of specific guidelines on FGM for schools and teachers. This therefore results in great uncertainties on how to best deal with cases of FGM that may become apparent.[5]

Many professionals are not equipped with the information and support required to effectively identify and deal with cases of FGM. This becomes of great concern, as they are often in a unique position to provide support, services and education due to the frequency with which they interact with practising communities. It is therefore imperative that robust measures are taken to educate and train HCPs and other authorities, on the social and cultural contexts of FGM, in order for these professionals to develop a culturally sensitive understanding of the practice and its harmful effects, and to then convey this to their patients or clients.

Training must also include effective protocols, detailing the procedure that specific professions must follow when a female is suspected to be at risk of FGM. Although organisations like FORWARD offer such inter-agency training, there is a lack of focused training, for specific professions, such as for midwives, doctors and teachers respectively.[21] This has been largely attributed to the lack of funding given towards the campaign against FGM.

Improving health and social services

The dichotomy in dealing with FGM lies in the need to prevent the practice, and to treat women who have been circumcised. FGM affects the physical, psychological, sexual and social well-being of women and girls. These problems must therefore not be forgotten, and, as such, there is a great need to enhance healthcare services for these women.

There are several Well Women Clinics in the UK that care specifically for women who have experienced genital mutilation. A specially trained team of health professionals runs them and they offer services such as specialist care during childbirth, de-infibulation ('reversals') and follow-up action with women and their families to provide education and information on the need to abolish the practice.[33] However, the lacunae in these services have been highlighted as salient points that must be addressed.

First, there is a need to increase the number of services which are available. In an interview with Comfort Momoh, she stated that there were too few clinics, most were concentrated in the south, and worked mainly on the basis of word of mouth. In some communities it is customary for infibulation to be reversed just before marriage, or immediately after, to facilitate consummation and subsequently childbirth.[33] This is often carried out by a birth attendant or a midwife, and thus facilitates consummation of the marriage. In the UK, however, many women find it difficult to obtain this service, as they either do not know that such services exist or they don't know how to access them. A direct corollary of this is that consummation is usually achieved solely by penile penetration, and therefore the vaginal opening remains too small for natural vaginal delivery.[34]

Second, services should be culturally accessible to women, with female staff and interpreters made increasingly available. This is in line with the cultural norms of many FGM-practising communities.[30] It is also important that cases of FGM are dealt with thoughtfully and sensitively. A qualitative study carried out in the urban areas of south Manchester surveyed women from the Sudanese and Somali communities. More than three-quarters of the women interviewed felt that significant improvements were needed in the health services in educating professionals, not only on FGM, but also on cultural sensitivity.[5]

In another qualitative survey of several Somali women who had undergone FGM, living in London, many expressed the desire that HCPs could be more knowledgeable about their culture.[26] One woman stated that 'it is immediately obvious that the doctor and nurses attitude towards you change immediately once they've discovered you've been cut … to disgust and horror'.[26]

According to Faduma Hassan, a Somali activist campaigning against FGM, due to the disparities in culture, Somali women who have been infibulated often have difficulties talking to Western women, as they feel 'Western health professionals are unable to understand their traditions and customs'.[25] This places a cultural barrier between the professional and the client. It may thus be important to involve circumcised women in the healthcare system, and train professionals about FGM and the reasons why it is practised. By using an approach sensitive to the beliefs and culture of particular communities, the effectiveness of caring for FGM 'sufferers' will be considerably improved.[30]

Third, services in place must be improved to augment the delivery of health and social care to women with FGM. This point is illustrated by a survey carried out in

2000 on the knowledge, attitudes and practices of health professionals in London. Of the HCPs interviewed, 78% felt they were not adequately prepared to manage the complications that may be associated with FGM, including psychological and psychosexual effects.[35]

Education and empowerment

The high regard that customs and traditions are often ascribed, and the fact that FGM is so deeply steeped in the cultures of communities which practise it, result in great difficulties trying to persuade a woman and her community to relinquish the practice. Drawing up legislations and policies is important, but the most arduous task lies in attempting to change behaviours and attitudes that have been embedded in societies and communities for decades. The abandonment of FGM necessitates the scaling up of efforts to educate and sensitise women, men and communities on the adverse effects of such a practice.

This is an act not only done by communities to the female, but an act done *by women to women*. Why do mothers continue to practise and surrender their daughters to the harmful effects of FGM that they themselves have experienced? The reasons for this are complex, and intricately located within a construct of patriarchal ideologies, issues of poverty and lack of education.

Gender can be defined as a social and cultural construct, determining the status, identity, roles and responsibilities of men and women.[36] Gender relations and the role of influences and power between men and women are therefore not static, but are historically, geographically and culturally specific. Societies and communities practising FGM are not homogenous. Gender relations and the status of women differ between cultures and families; however, several factors are common amongst practising ethnic groups in Africa in that women are often relegated to a position of subservience and dependence on men.[4]

This limited status results in women's lack of access to basic education and employment opportunities, thus disempowering them economically, politically and socially. This is a particularly potent issue when one considers empirical evidence on the lack of autonomy and decision making of women in communities where FGM is endemic.[37]

There has been increasing consensus within the literature that FGM can be explained in terms of the 'overarching patriarchal system' which exists in many practising communities.[38] As such, FGM is seen to represent one manifestation among many of the 'subjugation' of women within this system. Therefore gender must be put at the core of any analysis, which aims to address FGM.

As mentioned previously, in many of these communities an 'uncircumcised' woman is unlikely to find a man who will marry her. As such, FGM becomes a prerequisite for marriage. Their limited control and power over their lives consigns many of these women to a life where marriage and motherhood becomes the only route ensuring survival and a secure future.[7] Paradoxically, women who tightly guard and perpetuate the practice buttress this route. This is illustrated by the fact that women have a certain degree of control and influence in the midst of patriarchal settings, and in many FGM-practising communities this control is manifested through the 'circumcision' of daughters and granddaughters.[15]

In order for elimination campaigns to be successful, women from practising communities must be informed and educated, in a way that is sensitive to their culture and beliefs, on FGM's adverse effects. However, it has been empirically acknowledged that changes in knowledge do not necessarily equate to changes in behaviour.[39] Even when armed with knowledge, many of the poorest women will still find it difficult to break away from patriarchal ideologies so deeply embedded in their societies. Therefore women need to be given different means of empowerment, economically and socially, which does not necessitate giving up their sexual organs in return.[40]

It would be utopian to assume that once a woman is educated and empowered, achieving a greater degree of autonomy and decision-making power, the practice of FGM will automatically disappear. It has been argued, however, that if such initiatives were tightly coupled with greater access to culturally sensitive and neutral health education, as well as human rights education, then women would be better placed to make informed choices on whether or not to continue practising FGM.[41]

These women will be in an ideal position to disseminate their knowledge and experiences throughout their community, and thus play a crucial role in bringing about change. The employment of women from practising communities has been shown to be greatly effective, as many community members are sceptical of what they may perceive as an intrusion into their cultures by outsiders.[42] An example of this is Sally X who was circumcised in Senegal at the age of five, and now campaigns against the practice, as a peer educator for FORWARD.

She says both the experience of genital mutilation and her formal education has made her recognise that FGM is 'indeed a harmful practice; physically, psychologically, and mentally', and she is increasingly determined to ensure other girls 'do not suffer from this terrible act'.[26] She asserts that her campaign against FGM has been successful within her community, as there have 'been no circumcisions in (her) family since she was able to sit her father down, and tell him the experience of what she went through'.

Research has shown that women who have lived in the UK and have acculturated into the community are less likely to want to circumcise their own daughters.[43] In interviews with Somali women in London, many of them stated that they would 'never put (their) daughter through the pain (they) had endured'.[26]

However, many of them maintained that they would invariably be subjected to vigorous community and family pressures, especially by the older generation who fear that socialisation in a new community could lead to the loss of connection with tradition and culture.[33]

In the UK, it is becoming increasingly evident that community initiatives represent the major cornerstone for change, as it is these families and communities that must be educated first.[4] Such interventions are also more effective when there is a sense of ownership by women from the same communities, and that can also work to enhance their morale, self-esteem and motivation.[44]

Research has found that in many African communities, visual tools, such as dance, music and drama, are one of the most effective means of disseminating such information.[45] However, in educating communities on the dangers of FGM and the need for its elimination it is important to remember that communities are not static and work plans and programmes will need to be flexible to reflect this.

Although FGM is in a sphere which is dominated by women, the underlying realism of FGM is that women are circumcised *by women for men*. According to research by Black Women's Health and Family Support, young Somali men born in the United Kingdom said they did not mind if a Somali girl had not undergone FGM, but they also stated that they did not believe their mothers would allow them to marry 'such girls'.[46]

Any campaign to end FGM must include the education and sensitisation of men to increase their awareness of the practice and its physical and psychological consequences. There is also a need to target religious leaders and traditional leaders, who often demand a lot of respect and carry high influence within the community. The education of these leaders is important in endorsing to communities the fact that such practices are not required by religion or tradition, and they therefore have a central role to play in the campaign against FGM.

This is illustrated with the work of Pa Demba Diawara, a Senegalese imam who, after an educational programme on FGM with TOSTAN (a Senegal-based non-governmental organisation, working on the elimination of FGM), has worked extensively with his local community to abandon the practice:

> If I had known what I know now, I would have started 10 years ago.
> I did not know the amount of suffering our women had gone through.
> I did not know that the women in the village who were sterile had
> infections after their operation. I did not know that the girls who had
> died had died because of this practice ... We men never talked about it.
> We never asked and we just never knew.[41]

Due to its powerful channel of influence, the media can also play an important role in raising awareness within communities and in influencing public opinion. It has been suggested that the practice would decline dramatically if it was condemned by the media;[10] they should therefore be encouraged to feature items on FGM and its harmful effects. However, there is a danger that the media could over-sensationalise stories in order to create greater effects, and in so doing demonise the culture of practising communities. Therefore, in order to assist such campaign initiatives, governments, NGOs and other agencies working on FGM must ensure that materials are presented in a sensitive way, accurately and in conjunction with adequate explanation.[44]

FGM as a reason for seeking asylum

It has been argued that although, paradoxically, the 2003 Act claims to protect women from the threat of circumcision, women who have sought asylum in the UK for that very reason are more often than not systematically rejected.[47] Critics have maintained that until the British Government agrees to accept violence against women, including FGM, as grounds to seek asylum, 'it will continue to fail the girls it introduced the law (FGM Act 2003) to protect'.[47]

The production of gender guidelines for asylum case workers would bring the UK in line with other countries, including Canada, the United States of America and Australia, who have all produced guidelines which recognise that FGM may constitute persecution in particular circumstances.[48,49] According to the UNHCR, the failure or the unwillingness of authorities to provide protection for women who fear being compelled to undergo FGM themselves, or for their daughters, culminates in official acquiescence.[50] David Blunkett, former Home Secretary, has stated that in keeping in line with the 1951 UN Refugee Convention,* the British Government are willing to offer asylum to women:

> In circumstances where there is an escape from abuse, and where the state (of origin) itself is not providing adequate protection, we are not simply prepared to open floodgates, but are prepared to begin to look at each case openly and treat women sensitively.[16]

Therefore, asylum caseworkers and immigration and legal aid lawyers must be equipped with the adequate materials, such as accurate country-specific information on FGM, to deal with each asylum claim effectively.

Political commitment

It has been argued that the rhetoric around legislation against FGM is often much stronger than its implementation in practice. This was seen with the 1985 Act on female circumcision. As previously mentioned, critics argue that by passing a law, the Government concentrated on an initiative that cost them nothing financially. However, the responsibility for complementary actions, such as education and strategies for social change, is left largely under the onus of poorly funded and poorly resourced NGOs.[21]

As has been explicitly stated, the Government has a central role in tackling the issue of FGM in the UK. In order for legislation to be effective, the UK Government need to commit to all elements of the anti-FGM campaign. This includes positively assisting NGOs and others, campaigning against FGM with funding and other resources, crucial for the fortification and continuation of their work. Although a law which made FGM illegal in the UK was ratified almost 20 years ago, empirical data has shown that many people remain unaware of such legislation.[24]

The UK Government therefore has a responsibility for legislative education to the general public, communicating all the implications of the new law on FGM. In addition, the Government play a fundamental role in devising policies to ensure that effective information, training and guidance are given to the relevant authorities, including HCPs, refugee organisations and social and education services. In addition, ensuring that the relevant authorities are equipped with effective monitoring and reporting procedures to identify girls at risk of FGM, including those who have been taken abroad.

Robust efforts are needed from the international community, including the UK, to strengthen collaboration and co-operation with governments in countries where FGM is endemic. This will work to encourage national authorities and other

---

*The 1951 UN Refugee Convention defines a refugee as a person who 'owing to a well-founded fear of being persecuted for reasons of race, religion, nationality, membership in a particular social group' is outside their country of nationality and is unable to or, owing to such fear, is unwilling to avail himself of the protection of that country.

influential groups in such countries to develop mechanisms for the elimination of FGM, including legislation against FGM.

Research

Research is recognised as one of the most effective tools in policy-making and implementation. While there is extensive literature regarding the practice of FGM, there is a paucity of valid and reliable data and research on which to base effective policy decisions. There has been insufficient research on the prevalence, distribution and types of FGM worldwide, with current information derived from limited and fragmented data.[18] In the UK, there has been no comprehensive survey on the prevalence of FGM, and the distribution of ethnic minorities that practise it. There is a need to increase funding for such research initiatives, in order to devise and effectively carry out large-scale, accurate investigations of all aspects of FGM in the UK.

Dorkenoo has suggested that reliable and accurate data is needed on the incidence and recurrence rates of all types of FGM and its subsequent effects. She contends that descriptive research on the different forms of FGM, socio-demographic characteristics of practitioners, and other variables, such as the age of the girls that are genitally mutilated, are also important.[51] Such research is important in the identification of girls who may be at risk, and will thus be an important tool for HCPs and other relevant authorities.

The nature and degree of psychological and sexual damage is largely unexplored, and this information will be vital in developing the appropriate clinical support for those suffering from the reverberations of FGM.[1] Moreover, research is essential in properly assessing how social, cultural and religious values affect the behaviour of individuals and communities with regard to FGM, and thus discerning the most effective intervention strategies for FGM elimination.

Summary and recommendations

It would be naive to assume that FGM stops as soon as people from practising communities enter UK borders. Instead, evidence has shown that people migrating to a foreign country take their customs and traditions with them, and hold on to them very strongly. FGM is an issue which demands a collaborative approach, encompassing the involvement of, *inter alia*, the governments, NGOs, human rights activists, health professionals, teachers and social workers.[50]

The practice of FGM can be a life-threatening procedure that can damage a woman's physical and mental well-being. It is thus seen as a violation of a woman's rights to full bodily integrity and, as such, serious efforts must be made to ensure that the practice is discontinued and that interventions that aim to do this are successful. Any action that aims to eliminate FGM must take into account the multiplicity of factors that give rise to the practice. In order for legislation against FGM to be effective it must be coupled with other complementary action, such as proactive community education, strengthening of existing health and social services for FGM 'victims' and robust political commitment.

The following recommendations are presented to strengthen impetus to help those who are at risk of, or have undergone, genital mutilation, those who care for them, and to ensure the elimination of the practice.

1 Professionals

Healthcare professionals and other relevant professionals are in the best position to identify and monitor cases of FGM, and thus need to be trained and equipped with the appropriate information to carry out this task. It is recommended that:

- All key professionals (health, education, social workers, etc.) working with communities at risk must receive specific training on FGM and its associated risks.
- Professionals must act quickly and effectively when faced with an at-risk case of FGM. The girl must be placed on an at-risk register, and an experienced social worker put on the case. Focus should be preventative, educational and persuasive, and legal action should be the last resort.
- Specific guidance and training on FGM should be provided to schools and teachers. The Department for Education and Employment (DfEE) should develop materials on FGM for use in schools.

2 Health and social sector

FGM affects the physical, psychological and social well-being of many women and girls. Therefore proactive measures must be taken to improve the health and social services which will care for these women. It is recommended that:

- There needs to be an increase in the number of services caring for women who have undergone FGM, including protocols for de-infibulation, psychosexual and gynaecological help and individual and community counselling.
- FGM cases must be dealt with in a way that is sensitive to the woman's culture and beliefs.
- The Department of Health should set up a national helpline to offer confidential support and counselling for women who have undergone FGM.
- Adolescent girls who have undergone FGM should have special support services to deal with their specific needs.

3 Education and empowerment

FGM has been recognised as a gendered practice. As such, women need to be educated and empowered to make the decision not to continue the practice. Such initiatives must be coupled with the sensitisation and education of men and communities on the benefits of such change. It is recommended:

- Address the low status of women in many practising communities, through educational and empowerment programmes.
- Community education and empowerment programmes, sensitive to cultures and beliefs.
- Media campaigns should be implemented in order to raise awareness of the health and legal issues associated with FGM, and services and information available for communities.

4 Government commitment

Legislative action is only one component to an ideal solution of the FGM problem. The UK Government must address all aspects of FGM elimination campaigns. The following recommendations are made:

- The government must take a holistic approach in tackling FGM, and be active in drawing up legislation for FGM prevention and elimination, as well as in its implementation.
- The government must ensure that there are effective monitoring procedures in place for identifying girls at risk of FGM and protocols in place to protect them.
- The government should run a national campaign to convey the implications of the new law against FGM.
- The appropriate funding and support should be provided to NGOs working towards the elimination of FGM.
- Fear of gender-based violence, including FGM, should be widely seen as legitimate grounds to seek asylum and refugee status.

5 Research

Research is one of the most effective tools in policy and decision making. As such, there is a need for comprehensive studies on FGM to equip the UK government and organisations involved in FGM with a better understanding of the practice and effective strategies for its elimination. The following recommendations are made:

- Comprehensive surveys of the prevalence, incidence, distribution and types of FGM and their consequences should be carried out, worldwide and in the UK.
- Anthropological research should be carried out for greater understanding of FGM, in order to develop evidence-based elimination strategies.
- Research must be used effectively for the implementation of evidence-based interventions towards the elimination of FGM.

References

1 Royal College of General Practitioners (2001) *Female Genital Mutilation*. RCGP, London.
2 British Medical Association (2001) *Female Genital Mutilation: Caring for patients and child protection. Guidance from the British Medical Association*. BMA, London.
3 Abboud P, Quereux C, Mansour G *et al.* (2000) Stronger campaign needed to end female genital mutilation. *BMJ*. **320**: 1153.
4 Dorkenoo E (1995) *Cutting the Rose. Female genital mutilation: the practice and its prevention*. Minority Rights Publications, London.
5 Lockhat H (2004) *Female Genital Mutilation: treating the tears*. Middlesex University Press, London.
6 FORWARD (2001) *Strengthening Efforts to Stop Female Genital Mutilation: forum report*. Foundation for Women's Health Research and Development, London.
7 Lightfoot-Klein H and Shaw E (1991) Special needs of ritually circumcised women patients. *Journal of Obstetric, Gynaecologic and Neonatal Nursing*. **20**: 10–27.
8 Hedley R and Dorkenoo E (1992) *Child Protection and Female Genital Mutilation*. Foundation for Women's Health Research and Development, London.

9   World Health Organization (1996) *Female Genital Mutilation: report of a WHO technical working group*. WHO, Geneva.
10 Black JA and Debelle GD (1995) Female genital mutilation in Britain. *BMJ*. **310**: 1590–92.
11 Banda F (2003) National legislation against female genital mutilation. www.gtz.de (accessed 14 March 2004).
12 Amnesty International (2000) *Women's Rights are Human Rights: the struggle persists*. Amnesty International, London.
13 Shell-Duncan B (2001) The medicalisation of female 'circumcision': harm reduction or promotion of a dangerous practice? *Social Science and Medicine*. **52**: 1013–28.
14 WHO (1997) *Female Genital Mutilation: a joint WHO/UNICEF/UNFPA statement*. WHO, Geneva.
15 Toubia N (1995) *Female Genital Mutilation: a call for global action* (2e). Rainbo, New York.
16 Blunkett D (2004) Personal interview on female genital mutilation in the UK carried out on 3 March 2004 at FORWARD offices, Harrow.
17 WLUML (2004) *UK: Female Genital Mutilation Act 2003*. wluml.org/English/newsfulltxt.shtml (accessed 30 March 2004).
18 All Party Parliamentary Group on Population, Development and Health (APPG) (2000) *Parliamentary hearings on female genital mutilation*. APPG, England.
19 McCafferty C (2004) Personal interview on female genital mutilation, carried out on 26 February 2004 at the Houses of Parliament.
20 Momoh C (Midwife at specialist clinic in Guy's and St Thomas' hospitals) (2004) Personal interview on 'female genital mutilation and the role of health services and providers' on 13 April 2004 at Guy's and St Thomas' Hospitals, Waterloo.
21 Kwateng-Kluvitse A (Director, FORWARD) (2004) Personal interview on female genital mutilation, carried out on 3 April 2004 at FORWARD offices, Harrow.
22 Boyle E and Preves S (2000) National Politics as International Process: The Case of Anti-Female-Genital-Cutting Laws. *Law and Society Review*: **34**(3): 703–37.
23 Mohammad R (2003) *Culture and FGM* (unpublished paper). Foundation for Women's Health Research and Development.
24 All Party Parliamentary Group on Population, Development and Health (APPG) (2000) *Female genital mutilation. Survey report and analysis*. England: All Party Parliamentary Group on Population, Development and Reproductive Health.
25 Hassan Faduma (Black Women's Health & Family Support) (2004) Personal interview on female genital mutilation, carried out on 3 March 2004 at FORWARD offices, Harrow.
26 Anonymous (2004) Personal interviews with five Somali women who had undergone FGM on 'the experiences of female genital mutilation' held on 20 February 2004 in Brixton.
27 Royal College of Nursing (1996) *Female Genital Mutilation: the unspoken issue*. RCN, London.
28 Royal College of Midwives (1998) *Position Paper 21*. Royal College of Midwives, London.
29 RCGP (2001) *Female Genital Mutilation*. RCGP, London.
30 RCOG (2003) *Female Genital Mutilation*. Royal College of Obstetricians and Gynaecologists. www.rcog.org.uk/resources.pdf (accessed 27 March 2004).
31 Department of Health (DoH) (1999) *Working Together To Safeguard Children*. The Stationery Office, London.
32 BBC News Online (2004) Female circumcision act in force. www.bbc.co.uk (accessed 30 March 2004).
33 Momoh C (2003) *Female Genital Mutilation: information for health professionals*. King's Fund, London.
34 McCaffrey M, Jankowska A and Gordon H (1995) Management of female genital mutilation: the Northwick Park Hospital Experience. *British Journal of Obstetrics and Gynaecology*. **102**: 787–90.
35 Muanine E (2000) *Female Genital Mutilation: knowledge, attitudes and responses amongst communities and health professionals*. FORWARD, London.

36 Crawley H (2001) Gender, persecution and the concept of politics in the asylum determination process. *Forced Migration Review.* **9**: Gender and displacement.

37 Stromquist NP (1998) Roles and statuses of women. In: NP Stromquist *Women in the Third World: an encyclopaedia of contemporary issues.* Garland Publishing, New York & London.

38 Jones S (1999) *Female circumcision: towards a greater understanding.* Unpublished policy report.

39 Prochaska JO and DiClements C (1984) *The Transtheoretical Approach: crossing traditional foundations of change.* Irwin, Illinois.

40 Toubia N (2002) Eradicating violence against women and girls: strengthening efforts. 2–4 December 2002. International conference held in Berlin. www.gtz.de (accessed 30/2/2004).

41 FORWARD (2001) *Strengthening efforts to stop female genital mutilation: forum report.* Foundation for Women's Health Research and Development, London.

42 Celestine OC (2003) FGM: an insult on the dignity of women. *The Female Genital Cutting Education and Networking Project.* www.fgmnetwork.org (accessed 20 March 2004).

43 Department of Health (DoH 1998) *Experiences and views of young Somalis living in London on female circumcision.* The Stationery Office, London.

44 WHO (1996) *Female Genital Mutilation: information kit.* WHO, Geneva.

45 Lightfoot-Klein H (1989) *Prisoners of Ritual: an odyssey into Female Genital Mutilation in Africa.* The Haworth Press, New York.

46 Chaudry S (2004) Working to end female genital mutilation. *BMJ Career Focus.* **328**: 125.

47 RAINBO (2004) Press release on FGM. 3 March 2004. RAINBO, London.

48 Bashir L (1996) Female genital mutilation in the USA, an examination of criminal and asylum law. *American University Journal of Gender, Social Policy and Law.* **41**: 415–54.

49 Crawley H (1997) *Women as Asylums Seekers: a legal handbook.* Immigration Law Practitioners' Association and Refugee Action, London.

50 Amnesty International (1998) *Female Genital Mutilation: a human rights information pack.* Amnesty International, London.

51 Dorkenoo E (1996) Combating FGM: an agenda for the next decade. *World Health Statistics Quarterly.* **49**: 142–7.

Chapter Twelve

FGM: the next chapter in the struggle

Comfort Momoh

The practice of FGM is centuries old, steeped in tradition and ritualistic custom. Reasons given for its continuance are multiple and complex and until about 20 years ago it was performed under a veil of silence and secrecy. In the past, FGM was always seen as a health issue. That is because it was largely the medical fraternity who first saw the problems it caused – and because it was too sensitive: '… talking just about the health aspects was more acceptable'.

But Nahid Toubia points out that FGM is not a disease.

> It is something people do, which involves hearts, minds, beliefs, societies, religion, relationships between men and women – and between young and old. Thirty years of experience tells us that if you take a disease approach you will fail.

Many NGOs advocate a behavioural, social change approach to tackling the issues. Government policy can create an environment for change, they argued, while laws can help by empowering those who want to break social norms.[1]

Amongst some of the older generation of women in communities that practise FGM, they still hold firm to the notion that excision is a tradition that must be upheld and one that is non-negotiable, if their cultural heritage is to be preserved. The powerful influence of older women in perpetuating FGM should not be underestimated. It has to be remembered that in patriarchal societies, women have few opportunities to exert any power, so they hold on to what few aspects they can control.[2]

Despite religious leaders proclaiming that FGM has no religious basis, health professionals informing them of the harmful consequences, and youth workers, teachers and other respected members of these communities pointing out that a girl can be just as clean, pure and fertile after marriage; the older people, especially women, remain unconvinced.

It is worth reiterating that parents view FGM as an act of love; if they are not circumcised themselves, or they refuse to have their daughters circumcised, they believe that the family is condemning their daughter(s) to a life where they would be exposed to ridicule, social ostracism and one where men would view them as unfit for marriage and childbearing.

With the ever-increasing mobility of people around the world and the expansion of worldwide communication, access to information technology and 24-hour news coverage, the issue has become a topic of global discussion. With an increasing number of immigrants, asylum seekers and refugees coming to the West from Africa and the Middle East, for example, incidence of FGM in host countries persists.

The European Union (EU) has threatened to withdraw aid to countries that refuse to condemn or ban FGM, and 'turning a blind eye' is not considered a justifiable excuse for failing to act against FGM. In Britain and elsewhere, one can still find practitioners willing to perform FGM for the right price, despite legislation prohibiting the practice in most nations of the world. In 2004, UK legislation has been enacted to prevent children being taken abroad on the pretext of 'going on holiday' to undergo FGM.[3]

Box 12.1

My two sisters, myself and our mother went to visit our family back home. I assumed we were going for a holiday. A bit later they told us that we were going to be infibulated. The day before our operation was due to take place, another girl was infibulated and she died because of the operation. We were so scared and didn't want to suffer the same fate. But our parents told us it was an obligation, so we went. We fought back; we really thought we were going to die because of the pain. You have one woman holding your mouth so you won't scream, two holding your chest and the other two holding your legs. After we were infibulated, we had rope tied across our legs so it was like we had to learn to walk again. We had to try to go to the toilet, if you couldn't pass water in the next 10 days something was wrong. We were lucky, I suppose, we gradually recovered and didn't die like the other girl. But the memory and the pain never really goes.

A young woman of 22 tells us that she was infibulated
at the age of 8 (WHO)

Change can be a long, slow process. However, activists, non-governmental organisations (NGOs) and networks worldwide are working tirelessly to eradicate the practice of FGM and are making a valuable contribution to keeping the issue of FGM at the forefront of international debate on women's health and human rights. Over the last 20 years there has been a considerable number of measures and approaches introduced to eliminate FGM. Strategies have been innovative and varied, targeting specific groups or instigating campaigns to raise awareness of FGM and its harmful consequences.

In 1998, the World Health Organization stated:

> It is now possible to believe that the beginning of the end of female genital mutilation is here. Women in Africa and elsewhere, perhaps for the first time ever, have a serious chance of abolishing this humiliating practice while at the same time addressing other problems of discrimination and inequality that they face. With the right approaches locally and sensitive international support, female genital mutilation can and will be defeated.[4]

The goal of campaigners in Africa is to eradicate harmful traditional practices by 2010, but to achieve this monumental task there has to be a zero-tolerance approach to combat FGM.[5] In Burkina Faso, Nigeria, Mali, Djibouti and Guinea, the wives of these nations' presidents have added their voices to others in urging an end to the practice of FGM.[6] However, in Somalia, about 98% of women are estimated as having undergone FGM and it is almost as widespread in Ethiopia. NGOs have a wealth of experience in tackling FGM. They have learnt new and imaginative ways of drawing attention to the medical complications caused by FGM.

As men remain the decision-makers in many societies, educational sessions are held for men too. Most are spreading a broader message about sexual and reproductive health and addressing issues including HIV/AIDS, the risks of unprotected sex, family planning and safe childbirth. This has proved more successful than informing men and women about FGM in isolation.

There have been encouraging signs that politicians, religious leaders and local men with influence and status in the communities practising FGM are stepping forward and leading by example through their refusal to have their girl children circumcised. One worker in Mali sees the health approach as important, arguing that if more people could be convinced of the harmful aspects of FGM, the socio-cultural change will eventually follow.

Women's groups can help monitor progress made in eradicating FGM, support health education, promotion and protection of the health and well-being of women and girls and help facilitate work being done, thus empowering women to take a lead and do it for themselves. WOMANKIND Worldwide develops practical programmes in partnership with local, regional and national groups to tackle women's inequality in many of the world's poorest places. Those projects work to unlock women's potential and maximise their ability to make decisions about their own lives and the lives of their families, as well as contribute to the future of their community and country. In addition, they challenge the unacceptably high level of violence against women globally.

International organisations have made the eradication of FGM one of their main objectives through their work in Africa. Ending FGM means challenging deeply held beliefs and longstanding traditions. International organisations are ensuring that prevention and due process, in the form of community education and law making, go hand in hand. Simply making FGM illegal and punishing those who carry out the practice is not enough, since it is inextricably bound up with livelihoods, community identification and women's status, and therefore a more holistic approach is taken.

NGOs such as the Black Women's Health and Family Support (BWHFS) have a history of good work spanning many years. As a result of the trust built up within communities maintaining FGM, there are many examples of projects that find alternatives to the practice, which retain the concept of awarding girls rite of passage into womanhood but which do not involve mutilation. One example, amongst many, is that instigated by BAFROW; they believe this work 'demonstrates the value of comprehensive, integrated, and collaborative approaches; and the need for long-term, uninterrupted relationships with the communities'.[7]

A small-scale survey, carried out by FORWARD,[8] among police officers and health, education and social services professionals in UK found that '45% knew of communities where FGM is practised, but around 70% said they didn't know how to deal with it.'

Professionals working in spheres that are likely to encounter cases of FGM, or children at risk of having FGM need to understand the socio-cultural needs and belief systems of this vulnerable group. It is important to educate and empower men and women within the practising communities and this requires sensitivity and awareness of what drives this practice. The younger generation of women should be targeted for education and training and in the UK there needs to be recruitment of social workers from the communities practising FGM.[9]

At this point, it would be pertinent to introduce Amina Ahmed, a Development Family Support Worker for the Agency for Culture and Change Management in Sheffield.

Box 12.2

My work involves raising awareness of the awful practice of female genital mutilation, to educate women and girls and explain to them that FGM is nothing but damaging to their health and genital organs and tissues. My colleagues and I, at work, try hard to inform of the consequences of the new law, which came into force in March 2004.

There were a lot of difficulties from the community, who saw our work as interfering with their proud culture and traditional beliefs. Working together we can inform and bring home to them the problems that can, and usually do, arise as a result of FGM.

As I am a part of the Somali community myself I am proud to be Somali and proud of my heritage and culture. We are a proud people who have many good strong values but we have this one practice, female genital mutilation, which causes pain and long-term suffering to girls and women. This practice has gone on for years, centuries in fact, and is deeply rooted in the community's way of life.

In my own experience, I remember that I was playing with my friends and enjoying a nice sunny day. Suddenly, my friends turned against me and said that they did not want to play with me because I was not done, or that I was unclean. I put pressure on my Mother to have myself done so that I could be like my friends. My Grandma and my Mother had often told me that one day I would be done, to look like everyone else so that I could get married and have children. I had believed them since it was common for girls to be done.

One day I remember I was wearing a beautiful colourful dress when my Mum called me. I was held by the strongest women who sat on my chest holding my legs and hands and leaving me breathless and motionless. There was an old woman who was holding a small bag containing what I saw were dirty old scissors, sharp knives, sewing thread and thorns. This woman was the circumciser; she had no medical training or experience and even her eyesight was poor. She cut me up, removed my clitoris and my precious genitals and put them in a bag and threw them away.

I remember the painful, harmful and deadly moments and I cried and screamed but could not escape. The scars, the pain and the health problems I suffered are still with me today and will never ever go away. This happened to every girl who went through it. I could not escape and was told afterwards not to discuss what had happened to me because it was for my own good, my secret, belief, and culture and for the dignity of our future and our family. I was told that everyone had this done to them.

Today, it is a different century and I am campaigning against FGM, whether it is done for dignity, belief, beauty or pleasure. I am fighting the practice to protect girls and women so they do not go through what I went through.

FGM is against the law, human rights, and is violence against girls and women. I beg the international community to work together and STOP this practice.

I would like to call upon the Government and those in power to provide the support and funding resources needed to help fight to eliminate the practice in the UK and abroad. I would like to request professionals not to shy away from raising issues or asking questions. It is the only way we can get the message across to communities who practise FGM.

I would like to thank our funders and everyone who supports us with our work and campaigns towards the elimination of FGM. I also thank my colleagues for their courage and bravery in standing up to a hostile community to continue the campaign.

Please take back the information with you and help us with our fight against FGM.

Thank you

Principles to consider when planning interventions

1   When planning interventions for the elimination of FGM, it is essential to have background knowledge of the distinctive features of the culture, values and beliefs of each community.
2   The particular perceptions of each community must be understood and respected before embarking on collaborative campaigns to modify or change people's personal perspective of FGM.
3   Actions taken to eradicate FGM should be integrated into existing health promotion, health education, child protection and community development strategies.
4   It may be useful to assimilate the topic of FGM into broader issues of women's empowerment, human rights and sexual and reproductive health; if one seeks to address FGM in isolation, this can cause misunderstanding or may be thought of as secondary to the priority of day-to-day survival.
5   Accepting that FGM is based on tradition, power inequities and compliance with the dictates of practising communities, it is crucial to develop dialogue and partnerships with religious leaders, traditional healers and those with power and influence within practising communities. This is more likely to be achieved where local men and women are recruited to negotiate; many communities perceive Western intervention as an attempt to discredit their culture and interference by Westerners in issues that are not their concern.
6   Whilst terminology used in the West – for example, FGM – is widely used, this may not be understood or, worse, may be highly offensive to practising communities. Many of those continuing FGM cannot grasp the notion that

some consider FGM to be child abuse, and any campaign must first acknowledge that from communities' viewpoint FGM is an act of love.

7   National governments and international organisations must adopt clear
    policies and protocols for abolishing FGM, including enactment of legislation
    prohibiting the practice.

8   Research must continue into all aspects of FGM, including the incidence,
    prevalence, main reasons why FGM continues to be practised, and health
    consequences as well as operations research in order to support the design of
    appropriate interventions for eliminating it.

9   Utilise all channels of communication to inform target population; explore
    the literature on culturally sensitive media outlets that use drama, popular
    music and dance, for instance, to learn from such projects the most successful
    ways forward.

10 Medicalisation of FGM in any form is not acceptable and should be
    challenged where identified.

11 One-to-one counselling, outreach and specialist services should be expanded
    and advertised so that clients know where to access services.

12 Traditional healers and attendants must be retrained.

13 Harness innovation; alternative rites of passage for young girls should be
    encouraged.

14 Target young people and couples, in particular, and provide information
    holding unmutilated girls and women in high esteem, providing the neces-
    sary support to enable them to resist pressures to expose their daughters to
    FGM. Generally, young people are in the vanguard in creating new social
    norms but, at the same time, there is a need for sensitivity when working
    with young women who have already undergone FGM.

15 Enlist men's participation.

16 The health consequences of FGM, particularly regarding childbirth, should be
    highlighted.[10]

There is real and justifiable cause for optimism, evidenced in global action to
eradicate FGM. However, it has to be remembered that there are dangers to being
reactive, and the temptation to rush-through ill-conceived strategies in one's
determination to get the job done will, most likely, result in alienating those who
perpetuate FGM.

Although this is the final chapter of the book, the journey is not yet complete;
hence the title. Whilst it is usual to use the term conclusion, it is suggestive of a
door closing and the message throughout this book is: 'work in progress'. 'FGM:
the next chapter in the struggle' ends with an inspiring story of a couple in
Ethiopia ...

When saying 'I do' means saying 'I don't'

Abinet Aseffa

An Ethiopian bride and groom made international headlines by adding a
startling new pledge to their marriage vows. Now their courageous move
has made them Ethiopian role models.

At their Sept 2002 wedding in Durame, capital of Kembata district, 22-year-old bride Genet Girma wore a placard around her neck which declared: 'I am not circumcised, learn from me'.

Twenty-four-year-old Adissie Abossie's placard reciprocated: 'I am proud to marry an uncircumcised woman'.

Just how brave Girma and Abossie were in deciding to celebrate their marriage by taking a public stand against the practice of female genital mutilation (FGM) is hard to appreciate without some idea of how widespread the practice is.

The practice affects about 90% of the female population among all religious and ethnic groups in Ethiopia. It is performed on infants in the first week of life, as late as a few days before a woman's wedding, or during childhood or puberty.

But attitudes to FGM in Ethiopia and elsewhere are slowly changing due to government and non-governmental interventions. The Kembata Women's Self-Help Centre (KMG), for instance, has been quietly working to eradicate FGM since 1997 by educating young girls and their families about its dangers.

Its school and community-based workshops and individual follow-ups have led some 4000 women and girls in the Kembata region, 416 km south of the capital Addis Ababa, to sign a pledge against FGM — and Girma was one of them.

'The reason I was able to avoid being circumcised is because of the training I took through KMG,' says Girma, who persuaded her parents to delay the procedure. Another incentive was her fiancé's strong opposition. 'He told me that if I am circumcised he wouldn't marry me,' she adds.

Once she announced her engagement — still fearful that her parents would insist on the operation — Girma left her family home and lived with Abossie before the marriage.

Abossie knew from personal experience the suffering FGM causes. 'I was the first child and I could see how difficult [subsequent] deliveries were for my mother,' he explains. Women who have experienced the most extreme form of FGM must be cut open and resewn after every birth.

'After I understood that it resulted from circumcision, I decided not to marry a circumcised girl.'

The couple's decision to use their wedding as 'part of a campaign to eliminate FGM' initially alienated Girma's parents, who refused to attend the ceremony, fearing their uncircumcised daughter would bring shame on the family.

Nonetheless, some 2000 people turned up to celebrate the wedding, which was broadcast by Ethiopian television news, invited by the KMG.

Happily, Girma and her parents are now reconciled after they realised that instead of being ostracised, their daughter and son-in-law have become role models in Ethiopia.

Another dozen uncircumcised young women in Kembata and their husbands — all wearing placards around their necks — have since held anti-FGM weddings. When Genet Markos married, her family also couldn't accept her choice. The parents of her fiancé, Mulat Dutebcho, however, were very supportive. 'That is because,' says Dutebcho, 'my brother is chairperson for the advocacy services on FGM in the Hobichhaqqa area.' Dutebcho hopes to further influence his community by 'not letting our daughters be circumcised'.

KMG founder Dr Bogalech Gebre is thrilled, saying, 'every [anti-FGM] wedding is becoming a forum for education'. After Girma's and Abossie's marriage, Gebre accompanied the couple on a tour of other regions of Ethiopia where they shared their experiences with fellow anti-FGM campaigners.

Gebre acknowledges that what works in one community may not be appropriate for others. 'Change must come from within,' she notes. Many activists now believe that dialogue and education are more effective than top-down 'we-know-what's-best' directives against FGM – which can backfire and drive the practice underground.

Gebre, who was cut at the age of six, has said: 'I understood the purpose [of] female genital excision was to excise my mind, excise my ability to live with all my senses intact.'

Radhika Coomaraswamy, UN Special Rapporteur on Violence Against Women, agrees that FGM '… is related to the denial of sexual freedom for women.' A report by the UN Human Rights Commission launched in April says governments have made progress in enacting laws to protect women from FGM. However, criminalising the practice alone will not eliminate it.

'We have to devise creative kinds of strategies to deal with the issue.'

One girl child most definitely not at risk is Girma's and Abossie's two-month-old daughter. She is called Wimma, which means 'full' or 'complete'.

www.panos.org.uk

References

1 Toubia N Dr (2001) Speaking at the 'Fight FGM' forum organised by Black Women's Family Health and Support (BWFHS).
2 Momoh C (2003) Female genital mutilation. In: C Squire (ed.) *The Social Context of Birth*. Radcliffe Medical Press, Oxford.
3 Female Genital Mutilation Act 2003. Enacted 2004.
4 World Health Organization (1998) *Female Genital Mutilation: an overview*. WHO, Geneva.
5 Ras-Work B (2004) The President of the Inter-African Committee on Traditional Practices (IAC) speaking in the Ethiopian capital, Addis Ababa.
6 Mitchell A (2004) *AFRICA: Focus on efforts to eradicate female genital mutilation*. IRIN.
7 The Foundation for Research on Women's Health Productivity and the Environment (BAFROW) (1999) *Evaluation of the Women's Health Programme with Focus on the Elimination of Female Genital Mutilation*. The Gambia. Email: bafrow@gamtel.gm.
8 FORWARD A small-scale survey, among police officers and health, education and social services professionals in UK referred to by Lawrence A (2001) Training Coordinator for FORWARD, speaking at the 'Fight FGM' forum organised by Black Women's Family Health and Support (BWFHS).
9 Rendell R Baroness, Patron of BWHFS (2001) speaking at the 'Fight FGM' forum.
10 Adapted from Principles of WHO (1996).

Glossary

Angurya cuts	Describes the scraping of the tissue around the vaginal opening.
Calculus formation	May develop due to menstrual debris or urinary deposits in the vagina or in the space behind the bridge of skin created when infibulation is performed.
Clitoridectomy	Excision of clitoris; practised in nineteenth-century Europe to treat an array of 'female ailments', such as insanity, masturbation ...
Clitoris	A small, erect body of the female genitalia, partially hidden by the labia. It is highly sensitive, and can be a source of sexual pleasure and female orgasm. It is homologous to the penis of the male.
De-infibulation	Surgical procedure to open up the closed vagina of FGM 3.
Dermoid cyst	A benign growth consisting of a fibrous wall lined with stratified epithelium. Results from embedding of the skin tissue into the scar created by FGM. Lubricating glands continue to secrete, forming sacs full of cheesy material (*See* 9, colour plate section). The cysts may grow to the size of an orange or bigger.
Designer vagina	Alterations made to the vagina (such as vaginal tightening or lifting of labia) for non-medical reasons.
Dysuria	Difficulty or pain in urination.
Excision	Removal of the clitoral hood with or without removal of part, or all, of the clitoris, as part of the harmful practice of female genital mutilation.
Fistulae	Vesico-vaginal or recto-vaginal; may form as the result of an injury during FGM, or due to de-infibulation or re-infibulation, intercourse or obstructed labour. Continuous leakage of urine and faeces can plague the woman all her life and turn her into a social outcast.
Gender	Culturally defined roles and responsibilities for females and males that are learned, may change over time, and vary among societies.
Gishiri cuts	Posterior (or backward) cuts from the vagina into the perineum, as an attempt to increase the vaginal outlet to relieve obstructed labour. They often result in vesico-vaginal fistulae and damage to the anal sphincter.
Human rights	Rights to which people are entitled simply because they are human beings, regardless of their nationality, race, ethnicity, gender or religion.

Infibulation	Type 3 – infibulation or Pharaonic circumcision – The third and most drastic type of FGM, consisting of the removal of the clitoris, the adjacent labia (majora and minora), and the joining of the scraped sides of the vulva across the vagina, where they are secured with thorns or sewn with catgut or thread. A small opening is kept to allow passage of urine and menstrual blood. It is called 'Pharaonic' as the operation, according to historic documents, was already recorded in ancient Egypt more than 2000 years ago in Pharaonic times.
Keloid formations	Result from wound healing with hard scar tissue. These considerably shrink the genital orifice with attendant consequences.
Labia majora/minora	The folds of tissue lying on either side of the vaginal opening and forming the borders of the vulva. The labia minora (smaller, inside folds) protect the clitoris.
Masturbation	Sexual self-stimulation.
Neurinoma	Can develop where the dorsal nerve of the clitoris is cut. The whole genital area becomes permanently and unbearably painful.
Qu'ran (Koran)	Muslim Holy Book of the words of God revealed to the Prophet Mohamed
Re-infibulation	The re-suturing of Type 3 FGM, usually after childbirth.
Stenosis	Narrowing of a channel or opening.
Sunna	'Sunna' means 'tradition' in Arabic. Type 1 FGM.
TBA	Traditional Birth Attendant.
Zur-zur cuts	An incision made into the lip of the cervix in the hope of achieving vaginal delivery during prolonged or obstructive labour.

Useful addresses/contacts

Support services

The African Well Woman's Clinic
St Thomas' Hospital Trust
C/o Admin Office, 10th Floor North Wing, London SE1 9EH
Tel: 020 7188 6872
Mobile: 07956 542576
Pager: 08700555500 (Ask for 881018)
Email: Comfort.momoh@gstt.sthames.nhs.uk and cmomoh@hotmail.com
Contact: Comfort Momoh

The African Well Woman's Clinic was set up in September 1997 in response to an increasing number of women with FGM presenting at delivery suites and family planning clinics. The clinic provides counselling, advice, information and support to women with female circumcision and offers surgical de-infibulation where appropriate to pregnant and non-pregnant women. The clinic aims to perform antenatal reversals on pregnant women. The clinic is run by a full-time specialist midwife trained in public health and the care of women with FGM, and is supported by a female consultant (obstetrics and gynaecology).

African Well Woman's Clinic
Antenatal Clinic
Central Middlesex Hospital, Acton Lane, Park Royal, London NW10 7NS
Tel: 020 8965 5733
Contact: Mr Harry Gordon

African Women's Clinic
Women and Health, 4 Carol Street, Camden, London NW1 OHU
Tel: 020 7482 2786
Women can self-refer for services.

African Well Woman's Clinic
Northwick Park & St Mark's Hospitals, Watford Road, Harrow,
Middlesex HA1 3UJ
Tel: 020 8869 2880
Contact: Jeanette Carlsson

African Women's Health Clinic
Whittington Hospital, Level 5, Highgate Hill, London, N19 5NF
Tel: 020 7288 3482
Open last Wednesday of each month (afternoon only)
Home visits or women can attend the hospital clinic.
Contacts: Joy Clarke or Shamse Ahmed

Women's and Young People's Service
Sylvia Parkhurst Health Centre, Mile End Hospital, Bancrost Road,
London E1 4DG
Tel: 020 7377 7870
Open Monday–Friday 9am–5pm
Contact: Tammy Porter

African Women's Clinic
The Elizabeth Garret Anderson and Obstetric Hospital
Huntley Street, London WC1E 6DH
Tel: 020 7380 9773
Email: egappts@uclh.nhs.uk
Contact: Maligaye Bikoo

Agency for Culture and Change Management (ACCM)
11a Arundel Gate, Sheffield S1 2PN
Tel: 01142 750193
Email: smcculloch@accmsheffield.fsnet.co.uk

Akina Mama wa Afrika (AMwA)
334–336 Goswell Road, London EC1V 7LQ
Tel: 020 7713 5166
Fax: 020 7713 1959
Website: www.akinamama.org
Email: amwa@akinamama.org

AMwA is a Pan-African, non-governmental development organisation set up in
1985 by African women resident in the United Kingdom. The organisation, whose
name in Swahili means 'solidarity among African women', was founded as a forum
for African women to enable them to come together to discuss issues of concern
to them and to have their voices heard.

AMwA aims to develop services specifically for the benefit of African women.
It serves as a resource and research forum on issues affecting the lives of African
women today and provides a platform for them to participate in policy forming
and decision making. Through advocacy, the provision of information, networking
and training, AMwA focuses its attention on four main areas: community development, human rights, education and research, and international development.

As part of its Africa Programme, AMwA set up the African Women's Leadership Institute (AWLI) following the 4th UN World Conference on Women, held in
Beijing in 1995. AWLI is a regional training forum for women aged 25–40, the
aim of which is to foster critical thinking on gender issues, resource development
and strategic planning.

Birmingham Heartlands Hospital
Princess of Wales Women's Unit
Labour Ward, Bordesley Green East, Birmingham
Tel: 01214 243514
Contact: Alison Hughes or Teresa Ball

Black Women's Health and Family Support (BWHFS)
82 Russia Lane, Bethnal Green, London E2 9LU
Tel: 020 8980 3503
Email: bwhfs@btconnect.com

Black Women's Health and Family Support (BWHFS), an international non-governmental and community-based organisation, was established in 1982 by Shamis Dirir as a platform to bring black women together and work at grassroots level. BWHFS promotes the eradication of FGM, provides holistic care and supports grassroots projects, which support and empower women and their families in Britain and Africa, as well as influencing policymaking at the highest level. BWHFS differs from some other organisations working in the area of FGM in that they have direct contact with communities who practise FGM.

Community Health Project
Kirkdale House, 7 Kirkdale Road, London E11 1HP
Tel: 020 8928 2244
Contact: Jennifer Bourne/Faduma Hussein

Established in 1999 as the result of an identified need within the local population, as part of a team providing access to health for asylum seekers and refugees. Work with local community groups to raise awareness of the law and health complications of FGM.

Foundation for Women's Health Research & Development (FORWARD)
465–467 Harrow Road, London NW10 5NY
Tel: 020 8960 4000
Email: forward@forwarduk.org.uk

FORWARD is an international non-governmental organisation that aims to promote change, well-being and human dignity. FORWARD is dedicated to improving the health and well-being of African women and girls wherever they reside and promotes action to stop harmful traditional practices including early and forced marriages.

Global Consultant on Public Health: FGM & Surgical Reversals (GCPH)
10a Russell Gardens, Whetstone, London N20 0TR
Tel: 07956 407063
Email: comfort@fgmconsultancy.com
Website: www.fgmconsultancy.com

The GCPH FGM aims to have global action to highlight and address public health, reproductive health, sexual health and female genital mutilation (FGM) amongst professionals and the public, supporting and performing surgical reversal of FGM, to relieve women and girls of the complications. Supporting, educating and providing training to all professionals, globally, in order to raise awareness of the complications of FGM and teaching professionals how to be culturally sensitive when caring for women and girls who have undergone FGM.

Midlands Refugee Council
Eklas Ahmed
5th Floor, Smithfield House, Digbeth B5 6BS
Tel: 01212 422 200

Multicultural Antenatal Clinic
Liverpool Women's Hospital, Crown Street, Liverpool L8 755
Tel: 01517 089988
Contact: Dorcas Akeju

Chelsea and Westminster Hospital
Gynaecology and Midwifery Departments, 369 Fulham Road, London SW10 9NH
Tel: 020 8746 8000

St Mary's Hospital
Gynaecology and Midwifery Departments, Praed Street, London W2 1NY
Tel: 020 7886 6666

Research Action and Information Network for the Bodily Integrity of Women
(Rainb♀)
Suite 5a Queens Studios, 121 Salisbury Road, London NW6 6RG
Tel: 020 7625 3400
Email: info@rainbo.org

Rainb♀ is an African-led non-governmental organisation, established in 1994 and
working on issues of women's empowerment, gender, reproductive health, sexual
autonomy and freedom from violence, as central components of the African
development agenda.
    Rainb♀ specifically strives to enhance global efforts to eliminate the practice
of FGM through facilitating women's self-empowerment and accelerating social
change.

Women Being Concern International
K405 Tower Bridge Business Complex, 100 Clements Road, London SE16 4DG
Tel: 020 7740 1306
Email: ramat@womanbeing.org

Their main mission is to mobilise the grassroots communities towards achieving
sustainable development in Africa as well as other parts of the world where there
is need to improve the quality of life of disadvantaged people.

Useful contacts

EURONET (European Network for the Prevention of FGM in Europe)

In the past several years, Europe received many thousands of immigrants and
refugees from African countries practising female genital mutilation (FGM). As a

consequence, many NGOs, governments and professionals from various European countries developed initiatives to prevent this harmful traditional practice. At several occasions, the development of a non-African network was discussed:

- At the Fourth Regional Conference of the Inter-African Committee on Harmful Traditional Practices (November 1997) in Dakar. Mrs Nikki Denholm, a midwife from New Zealand, sent a first Newsletter to all the members who expressed the will to be part of this network. After this Newsletter, there was no follow-up.
- At the Second Study Conference on FGM in Göteborg (July 1998).
- At the FGM Expert Meeting in Ghent (November 1998).

Following the recommendations of the Göteborg Conference and the Ghent Expert Meeting, the International Centre for Reproductive Health (ICRH) took the initiative to write a project proposal, in order to get funding for establishing a network at European level. The project proposal on the Network was elaborated in close consultation with the Göteborg Group.

The project was approved and the network was initiated in December 1999. The networking project was co-ordinated by the International Centre for Reproductive Health (Ghent University, Belgium) and was carried out in partnership with the former Immigration Services Administration of the City of Göteborg. It finished end of November 2000.

To date (November 2004), EuroNet FGM has 25 members from 10 EU countries. EuroNet FGM aims at enhancing the health of immigrant women in Europe, in particular to fight FGM in Europe in a holistic approach. The Network believes that establishing co-operation at European level will be useful to avoid duplication of efforts, and to exchange experiences and information especially about resources, educational material, health material, good practices, databases, etc. EuroNet FGM is still very young and is currently searching for the necessary funds to become operational, but it has the potential to become the co-ordinating body at European level with regard to the prevention of FGM in Europe.

The Inter-African Committee (IAC)

The Inter-African Committee on Traditional Practices Affecting the Health of Women and Children is a non-governmental organisation working to promote the health of women and children in Africa by fighting harmful, and promoting beneficial, traditional practices.

IAC was created in 1984 at a seminar in Dakar to implement the recommendation made on the issues discussed: certain practices related to delivery; FGM; nutrition taboos and forced feeding of women; early childhood marriage; and the promotion of good traditional practices, such as breastfeeding and baby massage.

WOMANKIND Worldwide

Develops practical programmes in partnership with local, regional and national groups to tackle women's inequality in many of the world's poorest places. Those projects work to unlock women's potential and maximise their ability to make decisions about their own lives and the lives of their families, as well as contribute to the future of their community and country. Additionally, they challenge the unacceptably high level of violence against women globally.

WOMANKIND has made the eradication of FGM one of their main objectives through their work in East Africa. Ending FGM means challenging deeply held beliefs and longstanding traditions. WOMANKIND is ensuring that prevention and due process, in the form of community education and law making, go hand in hand. Simply making FGM illegal and punishing those who carry out the practice is not enough, since it is inextricably bound up with livelihoods, community identification and women's status, and therefore a more holistic approach is taken.

Women's National Congress (WNC)

WNC is the government's independent advisory body on women's issues, working in partnership with women's organisations representing up to 8 million women. The remit of WNC Violence Against Women Working Group (VAWWG), which is chaired by Nicola Harwin, is to develop a cohesive and effective voice to government on action needed to address violence against women.

The WNC VAWWG established a Female Genital Mutilation (FGM) Sub-group, chaired by Anne Weyman, Director of the Family Planning Association (FPA), and comprises representatives from specialist organisations in the field. It also has access to a much wider network of expertise and has regular contact with government officials, particularly within the Home Office (HO) and the Foreign and Commonwealth Office (FCO).

Throughout the progress of the FGM Act (2003) through Parliament, the WNC FGM Sub-group were extremely active, meeting regularly with the government officials responsible for drafting the Act and assisting with the drafting process. Following its enactment, members of the Group continued to meet with HO officials and some were awarded funding to raise awareness in the communities about the legislation. The Group continues to meet and work to ensure the effective utilisation of the Act and to protect young girls from FGM.

Index